—A MESSAGE FROM CHLOE—

"Dogs are NOT Cows"

By: Paul M. Willette, MD.

A MESSAGE FROM CHLOE: "DOGS ARE NOT COWS"

1405 SW 6th Avenue • Ocala, Florida 34471 • Phone 352-622-1825 • Fax 352-622-1875
Website: www.atlantic-pub.com • Email: sales@atlantic-pub.com
SAN Number: 268-1250

Library of Congress Control Number: 2020906417

Printed in the United States

PROJECT MANAGER: Kassandra White
INTERIOR LAYOUT AND JACKET DESIGN: Nicole Sturk

Table of Contents

Preface

A *Message from Chloe: Dogs are not Cows* is an important metaphor that dogs are carnivores that eat meat and bones (protein) and are not cows or herbivores that eat grass (carbohydrates). Chloe's message is that dog health starts with the appropriate diet and nutrition for a dog, namely a raw diet of meat or protein, as that is how the dog obtains its nutrition and energy for health. If we treat a dog's diet like a cow that eats mostly carbohydrates, a dog will have difficulty achieving health, longevity, and a good quality of life.

Chloe is a British Cream Golden Retriever that is friendly, smart, and loyal. Chloe's love is unconditional. Chloe cares about everyone that crosses her path. She communicates with facial expressions and body language, and without uttering a word any person is capable of knowing what she is saying. Chloe's day involves sleeping, eating meat with a bone, walking, and sprinting in the field. She is a free spirit. Chloe embodies health, and although she is getting older, she is gracefully aging in dog years.

Speaking of Chloe's health, what is good dog health? Better yet, what is dog health in general? I have to say, I wish I wrote this book when Chloe was a puppy. It took years for me to build the knowledge required to best take care of dogs, and while I have implemented many good things for her, writing this sooner could have made her life even better and made me a better dog owner. We can't think of dogs as seeing the world the same way humans do. They can smell in 3D; they have sensitive hearing, and they had lateral vision to track motion, which is a great for helping Chloe catch a tennis ball. Despite their movement capturing visions, dogs can't see all colors, such as green or red, as they only see blue and yellow. There's so much to know about dogs in order to help them live the healthiest life possible. Chloe says it's not too late; we are going to fight for quality of life and longevity for all dogs, making every day count. Chloe's wisdom will transcend time and help other dogs that she will never meet, but that's Chloe.

This book should be required reading for future, present, and past dog owners. How are dog different from humans? What diet is important? What is the impact of spaying and neutering? Read on to find out. Just like everything with Chloe, the message is usually profound, and it takes time to comprehend, but the sooner we learn from Chloe, the better Chloe's, and other dogs like her, health will be.

I hope you agree that reading *A Message from Chloe: "Dogs are not Cows"* is time well spent in improving dog's lives. As every owner knows, dogs enrich our own lives, so why wouldn't we want to give them the best care possible?

Author's Note

This book is designed to provide the reader with facts on dogs, their anatomy, and their health, pulled from my knowledge and several sources. Rather than provide the information in paragraphs of text, the layout is set up in a bullet point format, offering information in an easy to read way.

Chloe

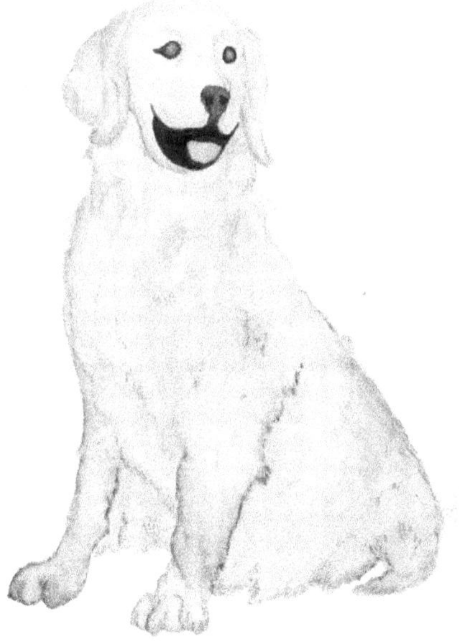

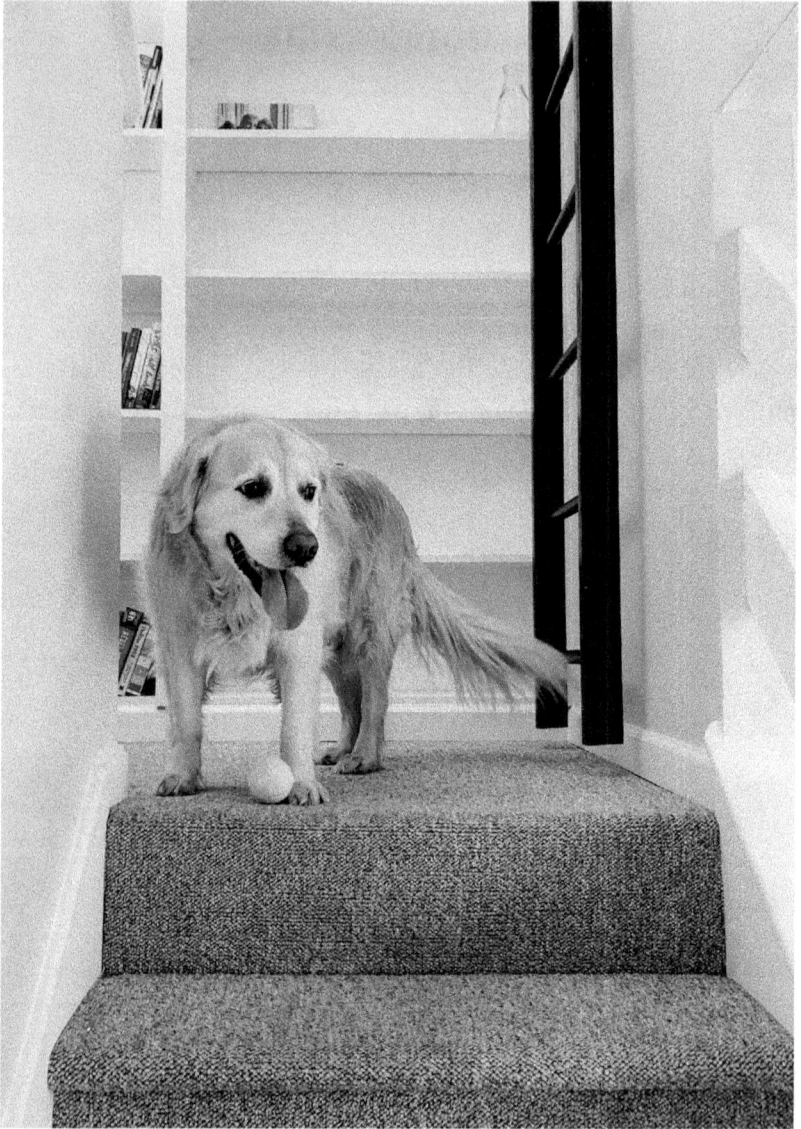

I. Dogs: In General

- Commonly referred to as "Man's Best Friend," dogs are one of the most popular pets in America and are generally known for their loyalty to their owners.
- There are nearly 70 million dogs in the United States.
- Nearly 1 in 3 households own a dog.
- "Most dogs love their masters (owners) 100 times more than their masters love them." [1]
- Nearly 1 million dogs are the main beneficiaries in their owner's last will.

1. Vinod, Ashwin, John Staughton, Rujuta Pradhan, and Salama Yusuf. "Why Are Dogs So Good At Smelling Things?" Science ABC, November 14, 2019. https://www.scienceabc.com/nature/animals/why-dogs-sense-of-smell-is-so-good.html.

II. Dogs: Their Head

- A dog's head, although it comes in many shapes and sizes, allows the dog as a carnivore to break up meat and bones with teeth and powerful jaws to swallow food in junks to be broken down by the acid in the stomach.
- The eyes, ears and nose are unique to each dog breed, but universal is the dog's keen sense of hearing and 3D smell.

Dogs: Their Head

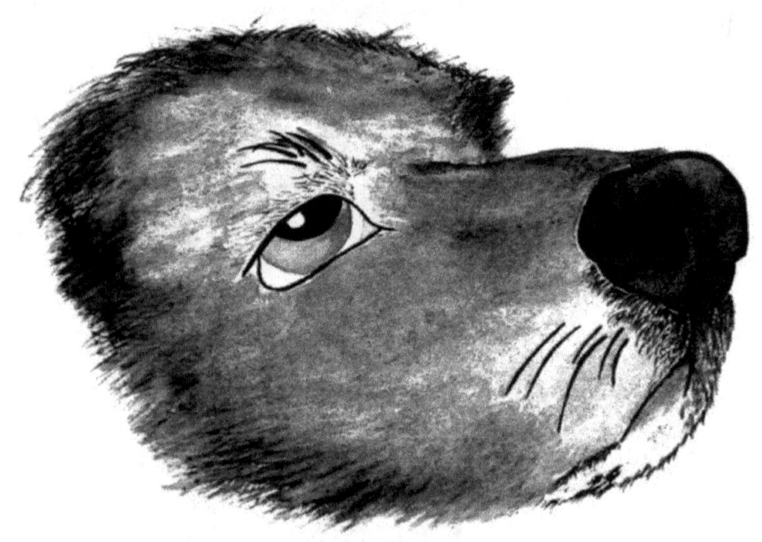

Jade Panyko

III. Dogs: Their Brain

- Dog brains are only one-tenth the size of a human's brain.[2]
- A dog's intelligence is on level with that of a 2-year-old human child; however, dogs do have skills no human could ever possess.[3]
- The dog's brain runs mainly on glucose, but it can use ketones during prolonged periods of fasting or not eating.
- A dog's brain has a much larger olfactory cortex than humans, about 40 times larger to be exact. Humans have a larger visual cortex than dogs, however.
  - The olfactory cortex processes the sense of smell; whereas, the visual cortex processes the visual information the brain receives
- "Proportionally, a dog's brain assigns 1.4X more space to analyzing smells than the human brain does." This mean that they have the capability to perform several tasks to assist people by:[4]
  - looking for lost or missing people.
  - using the power of their nose to help law enforcement detect drugs.
  - using their sense of smell to sniff for bombs with military and law enforcement personnel.
  - helping the handicapped or disadvantaged (therapy dogs, seeing eye dogs, etc.) use their smell and empathy as companions for those with stress and anxiety.

---

2. Foster, Bethney. "Facts About Dogs' Brains." Facts About Dogs' Brains | Dog Care - Daily Puppy, n.d. https://dogcare.dailypuppy.com/dogs-brains-2711.html.
3. Ibid.
4. Ibid.

Dogs: Their Brain

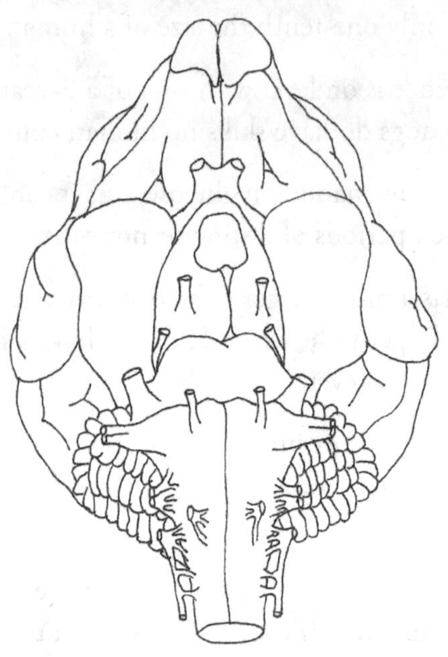

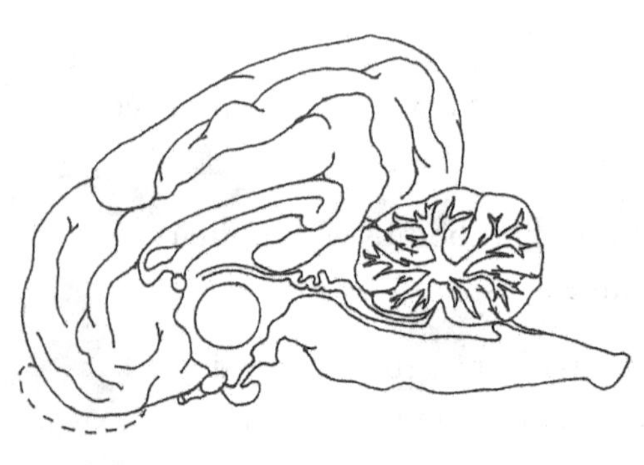

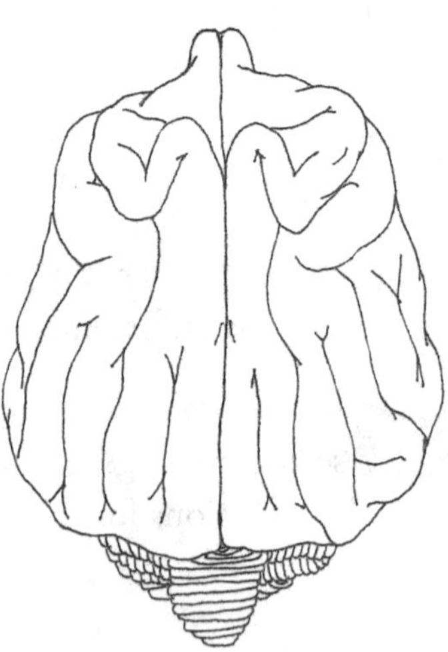

Jade Panyko

The Cerebral Cortex

- The cerebral cortex is the thought center for dogs' brains.
- " It produces learning, memory, empathy, behavior, attention, perceptual awareness, and problem-solving."[5]
- The cerebral cortex is divided into two hemispheres, the left and the right.
- The left hemisphere controls the dog's right side sensory and motor functions, even the tail wagging to the right, which denotes happiness.
- The right cerebral hemisphere controls the left side's sensory and motor functions, including the tail wagging to the left, which means a dog is aggressive or in a heightened state with the possibility of the dog acting with a fight or flight response.

The Limbic System

- The limbic system "is responsible for experiencing and expressing emotions, which can directly affect behavior."[6]
- The limbic system is associated with motivation, particularly as it relates to survival.
- The more important parts of the limbic system include the amygdala, the hippocampus, and the hypothalamus that are involved with fear, anger, hunger and sexual behavior.
- When it comes to a dog's behavior, the cerebral cortex and the limbic system are interrelated in dogs. Like in humans, changes in mood (anxiety or depression) or stress can impede the dog's ability to perform optimally.

---

5. Walden, Kat. "What Part of the Dog Brain Affects Behavior?" What Part of the Dog Brain Affects Behavior? | Dog Care - Daily Puppy, n.d. https://dogcare.dailypuppy.com/part-dog-brain-affects-behavior-5807.html.
6. Ibid.

The Amygdala

- The amygdala processes emotional reactions, both positive and negative.
- The amygdala is often associated with sensing anxiety and fear for survival purposes.
- The amygdala is also associated with repetitive behaviors and social interaction, and so it is more complex than previous thought.

The Hippocampus

- The hippocampus controls a dog's short-term memory and spatial navigation.
- Unlike the hippocampus in humans, a dog's hippocampus does not control their long-term memory, as long-term memory is mostly absent in canines.
- The hippocampus continues through the fornix as it communicates and ends in close proximity to the hypothalamus.

The Hypothalamus

- The hypothalamus integrates and coordinates chemical signals to the body related to thirst, hunger, reproduction, and the fight or flight response.
- The hypothalamus helps regulate the endocrine system because of its close connection with the pituitary gland.
- The hypothalamus also helps regulate the autonomic nervous system, which consists of 2 main components: the sympathetic system involved in a fight or flight response and a parasympathetic system used for rest, digestion, and repair.

- The hypothalamus helps regulate body temperature and the sleep/ wake cycle in response to light.

The Autonomic Nervous System

- The autonomic nervous system in dogs is divided into 2 major systems: the sympathetic and parasympathetic nervous system.
- The sympathetic nervous system is involved in expending energy in a "fight or flight" response, which is a generalized response to alarming or threatening situations that involves with increasing the body to act. The primary organs involved include: brain, heart, and lungs and the muscles that involve thinking whether to run or fight.
- The sympathetic system involves the thoracic and lumbar aspects of the spinal cord and is made up of preganglionic fibers that secrete acetylcholine and postganglionic fibers, which secrete norepinephrine. There is one main exception where the sympathetic fibers travel from the spinal cord direct to the adrenal medulla that primarily releases epinephrine into the blood stream.
- The parasympathetic nervous system regulates autonomic processes in the body, like digestion, heart rate, and respiration. The parasympathetic nervous system is generally involved with energy conservation and digestion, plus the elimination of waste products from the body.
- The parasympathetic system is often referred to the as the "rest, digest and repair system," which is an over simplification as the parasympathetic system does much more.
- The parasympathetic system originates in the brainstem and the sacral area or lower part of the spinal cord. The parasympathetic ganglia are present near or within the organs they supply. The pre and postganglionic parasympathetic nerve fibers secrete acetylcholine.

- The preganglionic fibers in the brainstem travel with the following head and neck cranial nerves: the oculomotor (CN3), facial (CN 7) and the glossopharyngeal (CN 9). The vagus nerves (CN10) and preganglionic parasympathetic fibers provide organs in thorax and abdomen. The sacral parasympathetic preganglionic nerves become the pelvic nerves innervating the structures of the pelvis.

IV. Dog Brain Neurotransmitters

- Neurotransmitters are chemicals in the brain that are used to communicate information from the brain to the body and vice versa. Neurochemicals work by stimulating or inhibiting the activity of cells in the brain (called neurons).[7]
- It is thought that a depletion or an excessive number of neurotransmitters can contribute to abnormal behavior.
- The major neurotransmitters in the dog's brain parallel the human brain including These neurotransmitters include serotonin, dopamine, norepinephrine, acetylcholine, and glutamate and GABA.[8]
- Low or high levels of neurotransmitters can occur for many reasons. However, a deficiency or excess of nutrients and building blocks required for optimal dog brain health is an under recognized, yet common and reversible, problem.
- Dogs that may have increased acute or chronic stress may have abnormal levels of neurotransmitters, resulting in difficulty learning or making proper judgments about what is truly a threat when none exists. This contributes to them experiencing more anxiety than normal.

Serotonin

- Serotonin is associated with many functions: sleep-wake cycles, appetite, mood, and impulse control.
- "A depletion of serotonin has been linked with aggression across many species. However, increasing serotonin can only make a change in aggressive behavior if there are already low levels of serotonin."[9]

---

7. "Neurotransmitters Implicated in Dog Aggression." K9aggression.com, 2020. https://k9aggression.com/neurotranmitters-implicated-dog-aggression/?v=f24485ae434a.
8. Ibid.
9. Ibid.

- "Serotonergic neurons originate from raphé nuclei in the brain stem. The axons of serotonergic neurons originate in the in raphé nuclei of the brainstem, particularly the midbrain, and reach almost every other structure in the brain."[10]
- Increasing L-tryptophan, which occurs in meats like chicken and turkey, can increase serotonin in dogs.
- Serotonin normally is associated with mood, while dopamine says more, more, more. Serotonin balances dopamine; as a result, serotonin puts the brakes on dopamine to function, optimally modulating behavior, mood and motivation.

Dopamine

- Dopamine neurons make up less than 1% of all neurons in the brain.
- "The neural projections of the dopaminergic system originate from the Ventral Tegmental Area and from the Substantia Nigra of the midbrain of the brainstem."[11]
- Dopamine can have both inhibitory and stimulating effects.
- Dopamine is mostly associated with pleasure, and it can contribute to the mood, memory, and learning of a dog.
- Dopamine can also be associated with reward seeking behavior.
- "Dopamine can sometimes inadvertently enhance aggression as low dopamine may create a more impulsive or less restrained behavior."[12]

---

10. Narvaes, Rodrigo, and Rosa Maria Martins De Almeida. "Aggressive Behavior and Three Neurotransmitters: Dopamine, GABA, and Serotonin—A Review of the Last 10 Years." *Psychology & Neuroscience* 7, no. 4 (2014): 601–7. https://doi.org/10.3922/j.psns.2014.4.20.
11. Ibid.
12. Ibid.

- The dopaminergic system is activated when an offensive dog meets a defensive one.
  "Dopamine's involvement in the regulation of aggressive behavior might be associated with competitive motivation. Aggressive behavior arises when conflict occurs between two individuals, and interpretation of the confrontation as a fight for resources makes dopamine's involvement quite predictable, because of its role in the reward system."[13]

- Dopamine also plays a role in risk taking behavior, where "risk evaluation is based on the size of the reward that is implied in the risk." This also plays into the aggression of dogs, as the risk of aggression may be used to achieve a greater reward.[14]

- "Low amounts (of dopamine) are associated with depression, the inability to initiate movement, or the inability to remain motionless."[15]

- Releasing too much dopamine can contribute to repetitive, purposeless behaviors or habits.[16]

- The nigrostriatal pathway (substatia nigra to dorsal striatum), mesolimbic pathway (ventral tegmental area to nucleus accumbens), and meso-cortical pathway (ventral tegmental area to the cerebral cortex) are dopamine pathways that are activated for movement, mood, motivation, and problem solving in dogs, which is similar to humans. However, the major difference is that humans have more long-term learning and memory, as well as the ability to plan for the future.

---

13. Ibid.
14. Ibid.
15. "Neurotransmitters Implicated in Dog Aggression." K9aggression.com, 2020. https://k9aggression.com/neurotranmitters-implicated-dog-aggression/?v=f24485ae434a.
16. Ibid.

Norepinephrine

- Norepinephrine is mostly associated with arousal, alertness, and attention.
- The norepinephrine neurotransmitter is concentrated primarily in the brainstem, specifically in the pons and the medulla oblongata in the locus coeruleus.
- It is also present in the sympathetic autonomic nervous system and is used for a fight or flight response. [17] This is because it can be involved with body functions during increased activity, like elevated heart rate and blood pressure.

Acetylcholine

- Acetylcholine is used for a dog's memory, arousal, and attention.
- Acetylcholine is found in cholinergic neurons within the brain and is located in clusters around the basal forebrain and the brainstem.
- It is also a part of the parasympathetic nervous system that deals with a dog's rest, digestion, and repair.[18]
- Acetylcholine is also part of the sympathetic autonomic nervous system as it is released from the preganglionic sympathetic neurons during the fight or flight response.
- The effects of acetylcholine within the brain and the body depend on the type of acetylcholine receptor the acetylcholine binds to. The nicotinic acetylcholine receptor bound to acetylcholine generally results in excitation of the neuron. The other acetylcholine receptor, called metabotropic or muscarinic receptors, binds to acetylcholine

17. Ibid.
18. Ibid.

with either excitation or inhibition depending on the location of the receptor within the body.

- Acetylcholine binds to nicotinic acetylcholine receptors at neuromuscular junctions for muscle contraction and preganglionic sympathetic and parasympathetic autonomic nervous system, while postganglionic parasympathetic receptors are muscarinic acetylcholine receptors with various actions both stimulatory and inhibitory.

Glutamate and GABA

- Glutamate is found throughout the dog's brain.
- Glutamate stimulates the neurons and causes them to be "excitatory."
- GABA is also found throughout the dog's brain.
- GABA inhibits the neurons from transmitting. In fact, "γ-Aminobutyric acid (GABA) is the main inhibitory neurotransmitter."[19]
- Many brain mechanisms' actions are influenced by GABA neurons, as they are projected to almost all areas of the brain.
- Glutamate is like the "on switch" while GABA is like the "off switch"
- Around 80 percent of the blood flow to the brain is for the Glutamine-Glutamate- GABA neurotransmitter pathway of the dog's brain.

---

19. Narvaes, Rodrigo, and Rosa Maria Martins De Almeida. "Aggressive Behavior and Three Neurotransmitters: Dopamine, GABA, and Serotonin—A Review of the Last 10 Years." *Psychology & Neuroscience* 7, no. 4 (2014): 601–7. https://doi.org/10.3922/j.psns.2014.4.20.

V. Dog: Major Hormones

- A male dog's brain and body health are influenced and explained by the hormone testosterone and serotonin.
- A female dog's brain and body health are influenced and explained by the two hormones estrogen and progesterone.
- Hormones are chemical messengers that communicate primarily via the blood or circulatory system between cells from distant sites from each other in the brain and body.

Testosterone

- Testosterone has 2 surges in male dogs. In utero testosterone spikes and influences brain development and hard wires behaviors until the next testosterone spike around puberty.
- Testosterone starts to rise in male dogs between the ages of 4 to 6 months and peaks when male dogs become adolescents between 6 and 12 months.
- Masculine characteristics seen in male dogs due to their testosterone include, roaming in search of a mate, lifting leg to mark urine, mounting, and competition with other male dogs. These behaviors decrease with castration or neutering.
- There are long-term health risks (ie higher cortisol levels and hypothyroid) with lower testosterone levels at such a young age during the lifespan of the dog that can be detrimental to the aging dog. Dogs with decreased testosterone due to neutering can experience muscle weakness, muscle atrophy, and a lack of bone density in his back legs and spine.
- "Decreasing testosterone (castration or neutering of the male dog) will decrease aggressive behavior of the dog, but as always there is unintended consequences of low testosterone levels of the dog long term."[20]

---

20. Ibid.

➢ Testosterone in dogs is regulated by the hypothalamic-pituitary-gonadal (HPG) axis.

➢ When a male dog needs testosterone as an adolescent and young adult but has been neutered, then the brain (hypothalamus and pituitary) tries to stimulate the adrenal cortex to compensate, but this has unintended consequences, such as increasing cortisol, which is detrimental as chronic and long term exposure.

Estrogen

➢ Estrogen is a steroid hormone. It is used to carry "physiological messages to the body's organs and systems."[21]

➢ One main function of estrogen is to communicate with the uterus to grow and replace the lining for reproduction in female dogs.

➢ Estrogen also plays a role in bone restoration. "Estrogen is needed to maintain a proper rate of bone breakdown for stronger healthier bones long term."[22]

➢ Fat stores in female dogs can secrete estrogen that normally has a survival benefit for reproduction.

➢ Lower thyroid levels (active T3) equals slower metabolism, which means more fat stores;. During pregnancy these act as helpful energy stores for the developing fetus, but for a dog with their uterus and ovaries removed the potential benefit of the fat stores is absent and the extra weight is more detrimental to the joints.

---

21. "Estrogen and Progesterone: Two Hormones That Control a Woman's Life." TAYLOR MEDICAL WELLNESS, WEIGHT LOSS AND AESTHETIC GROUP, n.d. https://taylormedicalgroup.net/healthtopics/estrogen-and-progesterone
22. Ibid.

Progesterone

- Progesterone is produced in the ovaries after ovulation.
- Progesterone, like estrogen, is a steroid hormone that communicates with body organs.
- "It instructs the uterine lining to stop growing so that it might develop and mature in preparation for a possible pregnancy… (however) If there is no pregnancy, progesterone decreases and signals the beginning of menses."[23]
- "Progesterone also promotes normal cell death in the breast, which is important in the prevention of cancer."[24]
- Progesterone plays a role in bone health as it stimulates osteoblasts to make bone. A balance of progesterone and estrogen promotes strong healthy bones long term in both male and female dogs.
- Progesterone has anti-cancer properties as it can help with balancing estrogen.
- Progesterone has anti-inflammatory properties and is important for healthy brain health.[25] "In the brain, progesterone binds GABA receptors. These receptors decrease anxiety, insomnia, and depression. Progesterone is a natural antidepressant and prevents anxiety."[26]
- When a dog needs more cortisol, progesterone can be converted to cortisol; therefore, the normal protective effects of progesterone are lost regarding brain health, bone health, and anti-cancer protection.

---

23. Ibid.
24. Ibid.
25. Ibid.
26. Mirimi, Rona. "The Importance of Estrogen and Progesterone." Fertility Aware, February 24, 2020. https://fertilityaware.co.za/the-importance-of-estrogen-and-progesterone/.

Cortisol

- Cortisol is a steroid hormone that is manufactured in the adrenal glands and spread throughout the bloodstream. "Almost every cell contains receptors for cortisol and so cortisol can have lots of different actions depending on which sort of cells it is acting upon. "[27]
- "The secretion of cortisol is mainly controlled by three inter-communicating regions of the body; the hypothalamus in the brain, the pituitary gland and the adrenal gland. This is called the hypothalamic–pituitary–adrenal axis. When cortisol levels in the blood are low, a group of cells in a region of the brain called the hypothalamus releases corticotropin releasing hormone (CRH), which causes the pituitary gland to secrete another hormone, adrenocorticotropin hormone (ACTH) into the bloodstream".[28]
- Cortisol is a hormone in dogs that helps with several things, including stress, weight, infections and illnesses, and blood sugar levels.
- Cortisol is actually the primary stress hormone that increases glucose in the bloodstream, "enhances the brain's use of glucose, and increases the availability of substances that repair tissues."[29]
- As a response to stress or stressful situations, more cortisol is generated and released in the body. This is because it is a

27. Kerby, Justin. "When Is the Best Time to Drink Coffee? (According to Science)." Cave Social, November 28, 2018. https://www.cavesocial.com/the-best-time-to-drink-coffee-according-to-science/.
28. "Explore Hormones,Observation, Treatment Details from Idea Clinics." Idea Clinics, 2020. https://www.ideaclinics.com/hormones-section/.
29. Desai, Rajiv. "Dr Rajiv Desai." Dr Rajiv Desai THE STRESS Comments, November 1, 2011. http://drrajivdesaimd.com/2011/11/01/the-stress/comment-page-10/.

hormone that helps the body appropriately respond to a fight or flight response.[30]

- "Cortisol…curbs functions that would be nonessential (like digestion in the gastrointestinal tract) in a fight-or-flight situation."[31] The goal of cortisol is to produce glucose in the blood for the brain, heart, and lungs and the muscles to either fight or run.
- Cortisol levels in the blood of domesticated dogs are generally higher in the morning, paralleling their human owners day/ night cycle. However, the levels are reversed in wild dogs as cortisol levels are higher at night as the dogs in the wild prepare to hunt for food. [32]
- Increased cortisol inhibits gastrointestinal function as the parasympathetic system normally allowing for rest, digestion, and repair is lowered or malfunctioning, which may affect the intestinal barrier, cause leaky gut, and ultimately contribute to immune problems or increased risk of infection.
- Cushing's syndrome can develop in dogs as a direct result of too much cortisol exposure.
- The symptoms of high cortisol levels are rapid weight gain, a large upper body and slender legs, high blood pressure, a flushed or rounded face, dry and/or itchy skin, osteoporosis, muscle weakness, mood swings, and an increase in thirst and/or urination.[33]

---

30. "Explore Hormones,Observation, Treatment Details from Idea Clinics." Idea Clinics, 2020. https://www.ideaclinics.com/hormones-section/.
31. Desai, Rajiv. "Dr Rajiv Desai." Dr Rajiv Desai THE STRESS Comments, November 1, 2011. http://drrajivdesaimd.com/2011/11/01/the-stress/comment-page-10/.
32. Kerby, Justin. "When Is the Best Time to Drink Coffee? (According to Science)." Cave Social, November 28, 2018. https://www.cavesocial.com/the-best-time-to-drink-coffee-according-to-science/.
33. "Explore Hormones,Observation, Treatment Details from Idea Clinics." Idea Clinics, 2020. https://www.ideaclinics.com/hormones-section/.

- Cortisol also wears down bone and ligaments.
- Unfortunately, as dogs age, especially if they underwent neutering or spaying sterilization procedures early in life, they can develop high cortisol levels and subsequent low thyroid levels with corresponding complications. In this situation the root cause is unrecognized and only prompts interventions for the symptoms and rarely addresses the root causes.

Aldosterone

- Aldosterone is a steroid hormone produced in the adrenal glands.
- Aldosterone is a hormone secreted by the adrenal cortex of the adrenal gland, and its purpose is to send signals to the organs that regulate things like sodium, potassium, and blood pressure. For example, it can communicate with the kidneys how much sodium and water to retain while allowing potassium to be released in the urine.[34]
- "Dogs with high levels of aldosterone have a condition known as hyperaldosteronism, and this can be from the ACTH stimulating the adrenal cortex in an effort to raise the sex hormones (testosterone and estrogen) but in doing so aldosterone and cortisol are increased as unintended consequences."[35]
- Dogs with hyperaldosteronism may have high blood pressure, abnormal blood volume, and low potassium, as low potassium can cause muscle weakness and low energy.

34. "Test 1 A&P 2 ENDOCRINE & BLOOD." Quizlet, 2020. https://quizlet.com/333893352/test-1-ap-2-endocrine-blood-diagram/.
35. "Aldosterone." Aldosterone | Endocrine Society, 2020. https://www.hormone.org/your-health-and-hormones/glands-and-hormones-a-to-z/hormones/aldosterone.

VI. Brain and Body Interactions: Putting it All Together

- "When it comes to dog behavior, the cerebral cortex and the limbic system have an important relationship with each other."[36] Like in humans, changes in mood (anxiety or depression) or stress can impede the dog's ability to perform optimally or impede happiness and overall health.
- "There is a direct link between the limbic system including the hypothalamus and the autonomic nervous system, which allows emotions to modify physical traits. For example, a dog's hunger and thirst centers are suppressed when he feels sad or depressed, which is why many dogs won't eat or drink while their owners are gone."[37]
- The hypothalamus controls homeostasis and hormones. Homeostasis is the maintenance or balance in stability in dogs that can be achieved with the autonomic nervous system or through hormones.
- The anterior pituitary produces growth hormone for growth. FSH (Follicle Stimulating Hormone) is for development and reproduction. LH (Luteinizing Hormone) is for testosterone production and reproduction. ACTH (Adrenocorticotropin Hormone) is for stress and fear responses. TSH (thyroid stimulating hormone) is for healthy metabolism, and Prolactin is for milk production in females.
- The Posterior Pituitary is for oxytocin, childbirth and lactation, compassion, and social bonding.
- Finally, the ADH (Antidiuretic Hormone) increases urine output and regulates blood pressure.

---

36. Kat Walden, "What Part of the Dog Brain Affects Behavior?," Dog Care - Daily Puppy, November 16, 2016, https://dogcare.dailypuppy.com/part-dog-brain-affects-behavior-5807.html.
37. Ibid.

- "Generally, serotonin has an inhibitory action on aggressive behavior. Whenever the levels of serotonin were lower, the effects of dopamine both good or bad could predominate."[38]
- GABA and Serotonin are generally calming forces and inhibit aggression.
- In a confrontation between dogs or with a dog and something else, dopamine and serotonin levels increase in anticipation of the confrontation.
- Both dopamine and serotonin are involved in coping with stress.
- In male dogs, the low testosterone (no testes) or in female dogs low estrogen (no ovaries) results in a feedback mechanism in the brain, specifically the hypothalamus and anterior pituitary releasing ACTH (Adrenocorticotropic Hormone), to stimulate the Adrenal Cortex to increase DHEA that will in turn increase the testosterone or estrogen in the male or female dogs respectively. Said another way, when spaying or neutering dogs, the loss of the hormone production from this action causes the adrenal gland to work harder to produce the missing hormones.
- Dogs can become aggressive when there are high levels of both cortisol and testosterone, but the solution is not to eliminate these hormones in an effort to make your dog or pet less aggressive as the cortisol and testosterone are critical for short term and long term health.
- Progesterone can block aldosterone receptors. If aldosterone causes the dogs body to swell and retain water, progesterone will cause water loss and reduce swelling.[39]

---

38. Narvaes, Rodrigo, and Rosa Maria Martins De Almeida. "Aggressive Behavior and Three Neurotransmitters: Dopamine, GABA, and Serotonin—A Review of the Last 10 Years." *Psychology & Neuroscience* 7, no. 4 (2014): 601–7. https://doi.org/10.3922/j.psns.2014.4.20.
39. "Estrogen and Progesterone: Two Hormones That Control a Woman's Life." TAYLOR MEDICAL WELLNESS, WEIGHT LOSS AND AESTHETIC GROUP, n.d. https://taylormedicalgroup.net/healthtopics/estrogen-and-progesterone.

- "By decreasing thyroid-binding globulin, progesterone increases the activity of the thyroid hormone. The thyroid hormone increases metabolism and utilizes the fat stored under estrogen influence for energy. Normal progesterone levels are important for normal body composition. Low progesterone levels can lead to weight gain."[40]

40. Ibid.

VII. Dogs: Their Brain Functions

- Dogs have the brain capacity to learn how to count, understand around 150 words, and solve problems.[41]
- Dogs have the intelligence to devise and play tricks on humans, dogs, and other animals.[42]
- "In much the same realm as a baby understanding that its cry draws the attention of its parents, a dog also understands that a bark elicits a reaction from its owners."[43]
- Dogs have the ability to understand their name and come when they are called. However, they mostly react to and understand tones.
    - "Happy tones make a dog excited and playful, while angry tones make dogs feel sad or frightened. If there is fear in your voice, the dog may believe that you're being threatened and rush to protect you. Sharp tones of pain may prompt comforting behavior from the dog."[44]

---

41. "Dog Psychology – 10 Facts on How Your Dog's Mind Works." The Fabulous Dog Bed Company, May 17, 2018. https://www.thefabulousdogbedcompany.co.uk/blog/read_184273/dog-psychology-10-facts-on-how-your-dogs-mind-works.html.
42. Ibid.
43. Ibid.
44. Ibid.

VIII. Dogs: Their Ears

➤ There are different types of ears for different dogs, based on what they are used for.

Rosebud Ears

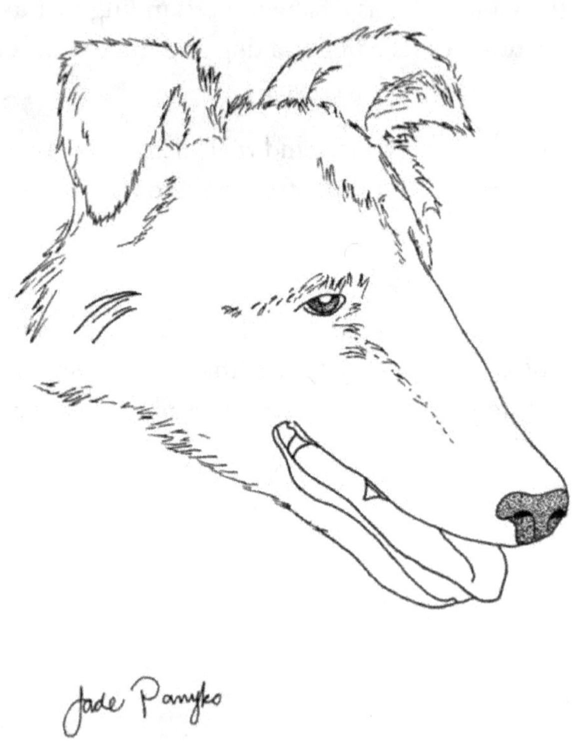

➤ Rosebud ears point upward and backwards. They are used both for speed, like in greyhounds, or for fighting, like in bull terriers. Rosebud ears are good for fighting because they are hard to bite

Drop Ears

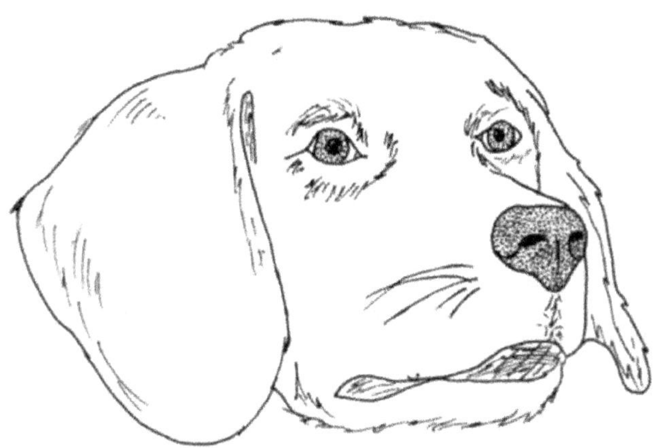

Jade Panyko

- Drop ears block out sound, so the dog can focus on smell. They are seen in dogs, such as bloodhounds, and are often referred to as "Floppy Ears."

Prick Ears

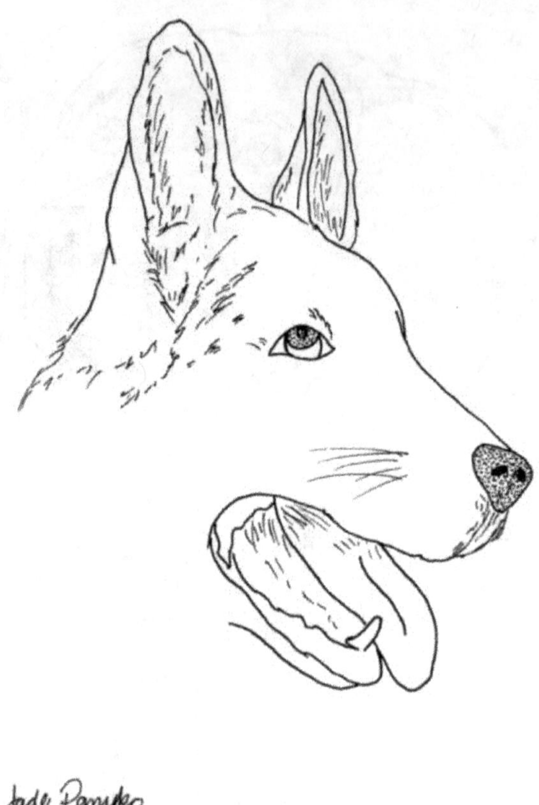

➤ Prick ears stand tall with a point at the end. They resemble the ears of wolves, and they are best for hearing because they can move to pick up sound or hear something specific. This is an extremely common ear in dogs and is seen in Siberian Huskies and German Shepherds.

Button Ears

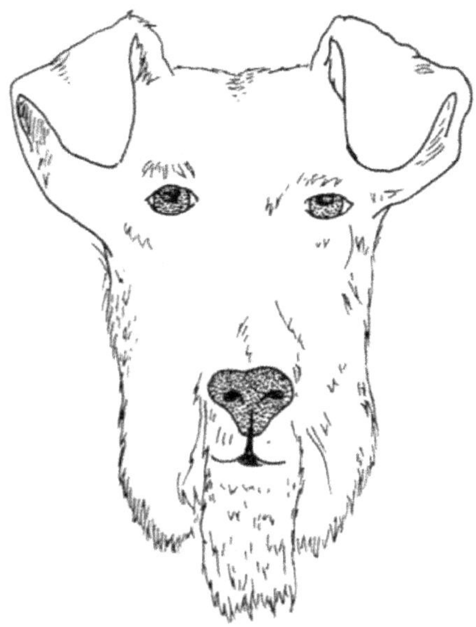

Jade Panyko

- Button ears start growing upwards then falls frontward. Breeds with these ears are Pugs and Fox Terriers. These ears help the dog crawl through a tunnel during hunting

Pendant Ears

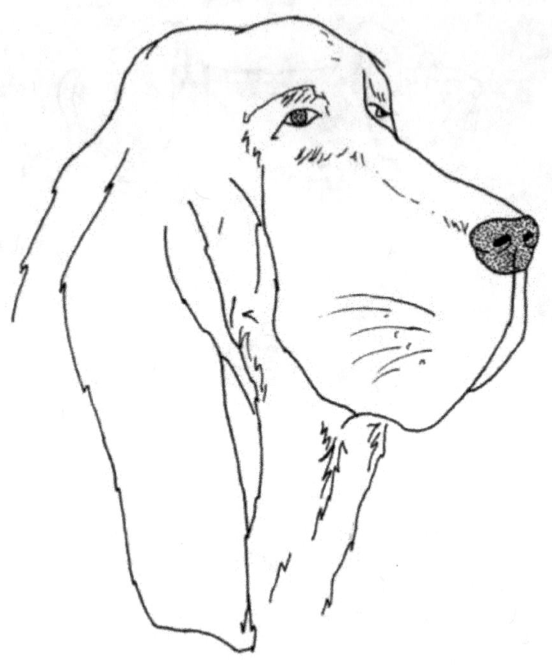

Jade Panyko

➤ Pendant ears hang down from where they are attached from the head. They are similar to Drop Ears. The Basset Hound is a good example of a dog with pendant ears.

IX. Dogs: Their Hearing

- Dogs have much more sensitive hearing than humans, hearing sounds that are four times farther away than humans.
- As dogs can hear only sounds and not words or human language, effective communication between a dog and their owner can be improved as the dog can pair sounds with actions in order to be able to understand and interpret what the sounds mean. Said another way, dog training involves the dog pairing actions with sounds.
- "They can hear higher frequency sounds, and can more easily differentiate sounds (e.g. they may recognize the sound of your car), and they can pin point the exact location of the sound."[45]

Why Can Dogs Hear Better Than Humans?

- Dogs control their ears with 18 muscles, but humans only have 6 muscles for their ears. Furthermore, humans can only move their ears a little, whereas "dogs can tilt and rotate their ears to funnel the sound into the inner ear more efficiently."[46]
- Dogs' ears, or many of them, are shaped to help them amplify the sound they hear. Humans' ears are not.
- "The canine ear canal is considerably longer than the human counterpart. Muscles allow it to finely tune the position of this inner ear canal so that it can localize a sound, hear it more accurately and from farther away."[47]

---

45. Kehoe, Siobhan. "Why Do Dogs Hear Better than Humans?" HeadStuff, March 31, 2015. https://www.headstuff.org/topical/science/dogs-hear-better-humans/.
46. Ibid.
47. Ibid.

X. Dogs: Their Eyes

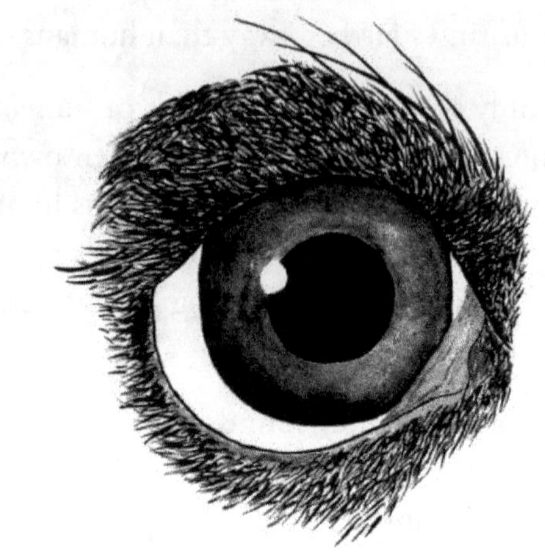

Jade Panyko

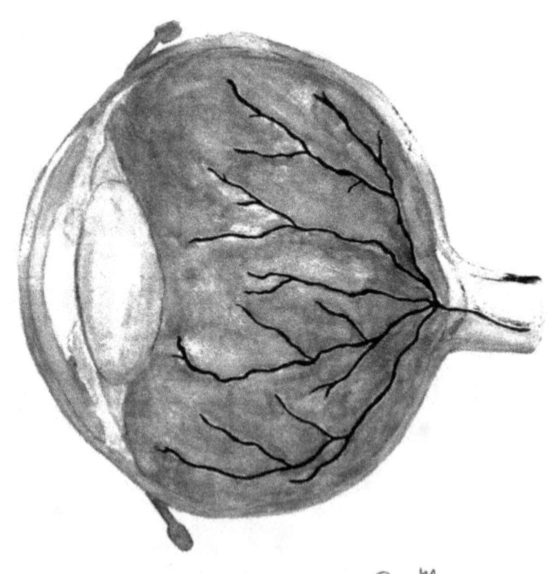

Jade Panyko

Dogs: Their Eyesight

- Dogs tend to be nearsighted
- Dogs' eyesight is 20/75. As a reference, in human vision the 20/20 vision is the ability to read at a certain level at 20 feet. Whatever a person can see at 75 feet is how well a dog sees at 20 feet. Its' not that the dog does not see at 20 feet; it is just a less clear or grainy picture. It's just like watching a television or computer screen with 75% less pixels, which makes the image fuzzier.
- Dogs' vision has receptors for color, called cones, and receptors, called rods, for black and white (gray).
- Dogs are able to distinguish shades of gray, but they less able to discern different levels of brightness compared to humans
- Dogs have 2 color receptors, blue and yellow. This is unlike humans whose 3 primary cone receptors are blue, green and red. This means that red and green may be indistinguishable for dogs, so if you are choosing a ball or toy for your dog, choose blue or yellow.
- The dog can see almost 5x the lower limit of the human eye, meaning they can see better than humans at lower levels of light or darkness. Dogs have enlarged pupils, which allows more light in and creates a higher density for the rods to process the lower level of light.
- Dogs are much more sensitive to motion at a distance 10-20x a human. Dogs' vision is most suitable for hunting at dawn and dusk.
- The visual acuity of the dog may be reduced, but the ability of a dog to detect movement even in low light conditions is exceptional.
- The dog's peripheral vision is 240 degrees, compared to the 180 degrees of a human. In their ancestors, the wolves, this makes them good at scanning the horizon for predators.

XI. Dogs: Their Noses

- Dogs use their nose to view and understand the world in the same way a human uses their eyes. Their sense of smell is the equivalent of a human's sense of sight.[48]
- Dog noses are wet for a specific reason. "The mucus on the dog's nose helps it smell by capturing scent particles."[49]
- When odors within the air are breathed into the nose, most air goes to the lungs, but some of the air goes to the olfactory recess, which creates more surface area with hundreds of millions of sensory cells that feed information to the brain.
- Dogs have 15x more sensory input than humans.
- As dogs sniff nearly 5x per second and sample the odors in the air, the dog inhales through front nostrils and exhales air through side slits of the nose, allowing sampling of the air with each inhalation. This is unlike humans who have to inhale and exhale from the same nostril area.

---

48. Vinod, Ashwin, John Staughton, Rujuta Pradhan, and Salama Yusuf. "Why Are Dogs So Good At Smelling Things?" Science ABC, November 14, 2019. https://www.scienceabc.com/nature/animals/why-dogs-sense-of-smell-is-so-good.html
49. Ibid.

The Nose

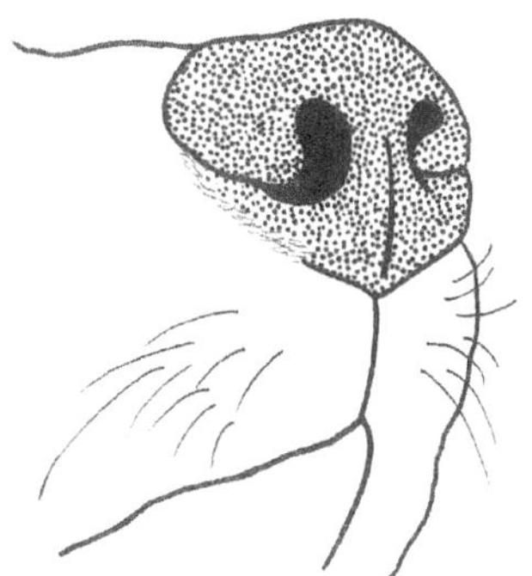

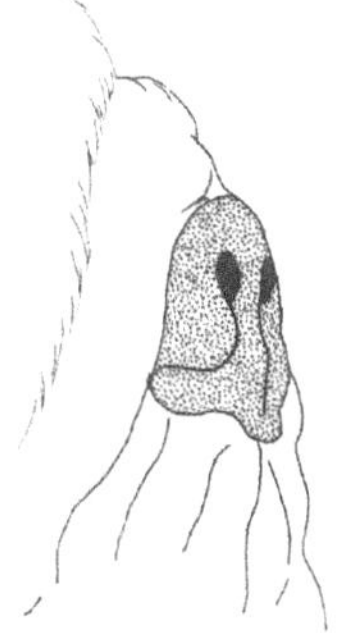

The Nostrils

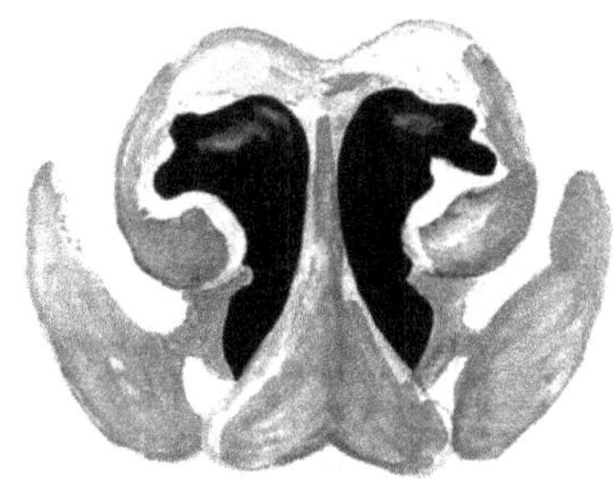

Dogs: Their Sense of Smell

- Dogs view the world most through their sense of smell. Furthermore, their sense of smell cannot be tricked.
- "Every smell is different for a dog, and each smell has a story behind it. When a dog smells a person, another dog, or any random scent, he is trying to determine the history behind it."[50]
- "A dog's sense of smell is far greater than a human's sense of smell." In fact, they can smell anywhere from 1,000-10,000 times better than humans. [51]
- Dogs smell in 3D.
- Dogs can independently smell out of each nostril. One reason for this is that is allow them to determine which direction a smell came from. "A dog's brain uses the different odor profiles from each nostril to determine exactly where smelly objects are in the environment."[52]
- Dogs have 225-300 million smell receptors, as opposed to the 5 million or so in humans. In effect, dogs have 50x the smell or olfactory receptors than humans.
- "The passage through which dogs smell the air contains highly specialized olfactory receptor cells, which are responsible for receiving smells."[53]
- The vomeronasal or Jacobson's organ is a special olfactory system located above the roof of their mouth. This "helps dogs sense things that they cannot see, such as human emotions. A dog can tell if a person is sad or happy, and this also helps dogs know whether an animal is friendly or dangerous to them. This unique ability also helps them identify potential mates."[54]

---

50. Ibid.
51. Ibid.
52. Ibid.
53. Ibid.
54. Ibid.

- The power of a dog's smell can be used to help humans in a variety of ways. Dogs can determine if someone is sick, detect if there are drugs or explosives, and sense the emotions of humans. "They can sense the emotions of humans and react appropriately in a time of need, and they also have been able to help in the early detection of cancer in humans, essentially saving the lives of their owners."[55]

- "The flight-or-fight hormone, adrenaline, is undetectable by our noses, but dogs can apparently smell it. In addition, fear or anxiety is often accompanied by increased heart rate and blood flow, which sends telltale body chemicals more quickly to the skin surface. Trying to mask your strong feelings with a casual smile may fool your friends, but it's not going to fool a dog's sense of smell."[56]

- Dogs use their smell to send messages through peeing. "Dogs read about the world through their noses, and they write their messages, at least to other dogs, in their urine." It's tempting to drag your dog along on a walk when he's sniffing everything annoyingly slowly, but give him chance to read the neighborhood gossip column, and let him do a little writing while he's at it.[57]

- But why do dogs smell each other's butts? Sniffing each other allows dogs to learn the history or each other. For examples they may be able to determine things like "Oh, you're a nice dog, and you had bone recently, and you're about, um, 7 years old?"[58]

---

55. Ibid.
56. Welch, Jeffrey. "7 Amazing Facts About Your Dog's Sense of Smell." 7 Amazing Facts About Your Dog's Sense of Smell, February 21, 2019. http://jeffreyrwelch.blogspot.com/2019/02/7-amazing-facts-about-your-dogs-sense.html.
57. Ibid.
58. Ibid.

XII. Dogs: Their Skeleton

- For heathy bones and a healthy skeleton, dogs need key minerals: calcium, magnesium, and Vitamin D3.
- A dog's acidity of the stomach can break down bones from their meal they consume (whether it's a T-bone steak or fresh kill in the wild), providing the minerals needed for their own bones.
- Healthy bone function requires constant remodeling, breakdown and build up, of new bone. Estrogen affects osteoclasts (breaks down bone) and progesterone affects osteoblasts (makes bone). The estrogen and progesterone need to be balanced for healthy bones. Testosterone even in male dogs is converted to estrogen as it is the estrogen and progesterone that is needed for healthy bones.

Dogs: Their Skeleton

Jade Panyko

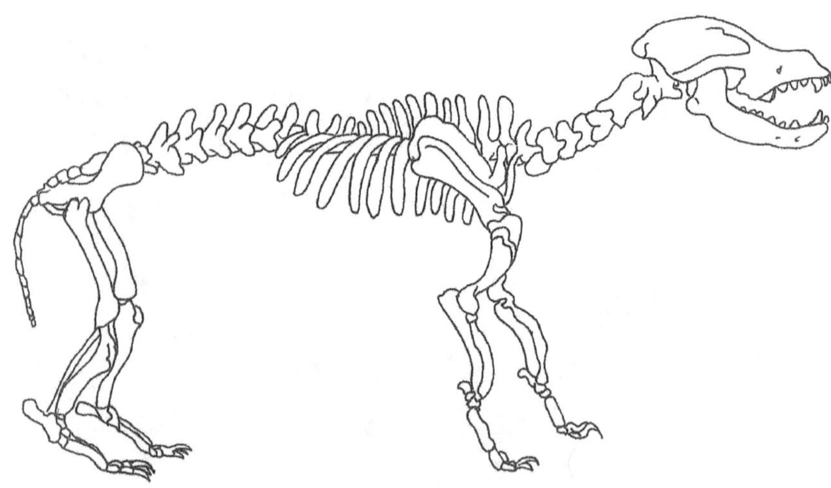

Dogs: Their Muscles

- Dogs' skeletal muscle reflects the diet and activity over the past 4 to 6 weeks as muscle is constantly broken down and rebuilt.
- The muscle health of a dog parallels other mammals and is not all that different than the muscles care of humans. The dog's muscle health is determined by diet and nutrition, exercise and hormonal balance.
- Dogs' skeletal muscle needs all essential amino acids to have the ability for muscle growth.
- Exercise and movement for dogs is good for the brain health of your dog's mood, happiness, and well-being.
- Glutamine is the most common amino acid in skeletal muscles and can be supplemented for muscle, as well as intestinal and immune health.
- Testosterone and growth hormones are helpful to build more muscle mass. Sprinting or other high-energy activity is needed in addition to low-level exercise or walking.
- The dog's muscles are a source of potential energy as skeletal muscle can atrophy when it is less developed and weak in strength due to the fact that calorie intake is lower in relation to the dog's daily energy needs for every day functioning independent of exercise. A stray dog or a sheltered dog may exhibit both muscle loss and weakness.
- A dog's poorly developed and impaired functioning muscle and joints can be from prolonged stress (physical, emotional, and hormonal) from chronic cortisol exposure that breaks down muscle and must be neutralized for stronger healthier muscles.
- It is important for dogs to walk regularly and have periods of running and sprinting as well.

➤ An over -weight dog can swim in a pool to exercise while keeping the joints healthy until the dog returns to a more normal baseline weight.

The Skeletal Muscle

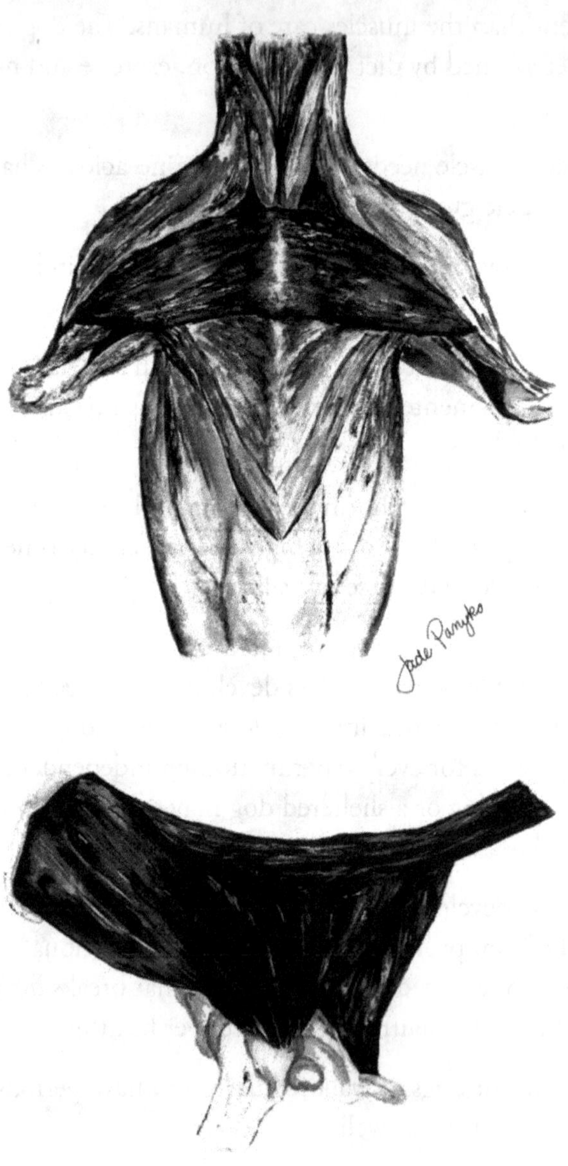

XIII. Dogs and Their Digestive System.

Their Teeth and Jaw

- The dog has a hinged jaw with canines, fangs, and incisors that collectively bite, hold, and pierce flesh in order to break up food into chunks that are swallowed down the esophagus to the stomach.
- Dogs do not have numerous molars for grinding food like omnivores and herbivores.
- The dog has no amylase in the salivary glands to break down plant materials like cellulose.
- The dog does have lysozymes in the saliva, however, that helps neutralize the bacterial load of the food even before it enters the stomach.

Their Stomach

- The gastric acidity (gastric PH) of the stomach of a dog eating a diet predominantly made up of raw meat has a very low PH of 2 or lower, which is highly acidic relative to the pH level of the meat or protein. "This highly acidic environment favors the breakdown of raw meats, and raw bones, into soft digestible material. The low PH also is highly effective at killing bacteria, particularly potentially pathogenic bacteria like Salmonella, Clostridia, Campylobacter and E Coli. So the natural 'wild' diet of dogs has evolved into a gastric environment that favors the breakdown of raw meats, raw bones, and a PH that kills potentially harmful bacteria – consistent with the requirements of carnivores, and in particular, the scavenging nature of dogs."[59]
- The acidity of the stomach is a powerful chemical defense barrier to infection, including bacteria, viruses and other pathogens.

---

59. Jasek, Judy. "FAQ's," February 19, 2020. https://rawdogfoodandco.com/transition-raw-dog-food/.

- Dogs lymphatic system parallels the gastrointestinal tract Mucosa Associated Lymphatic Tissue (MALT) as the outside world, such .as in humans. Food goes through the intestinal tract into the body. All animals, including dogs, are no different in that respect.
- The goal of a dogs stomach is to breakdown protein into polypeptide chains that are eventually further broken down to amino acids that can be absorbed as nutrition, while keeping pathogens or unhealth microbes out.
- Fresh and diverse foods are healthy for dogs. You do not need to cook your dog a hamburger, as the raw hamburger meat is just fine.
- Although the stomach is small, it is highly distensible allowing the dog to gorge as the acidity of the dog's stomach can break down bone hide and bacteria before it enters the small intestine.
- The dog is adept at vomiting if the volume or consistency of food is incompatible with the dog's digestive system.

Their Stomach

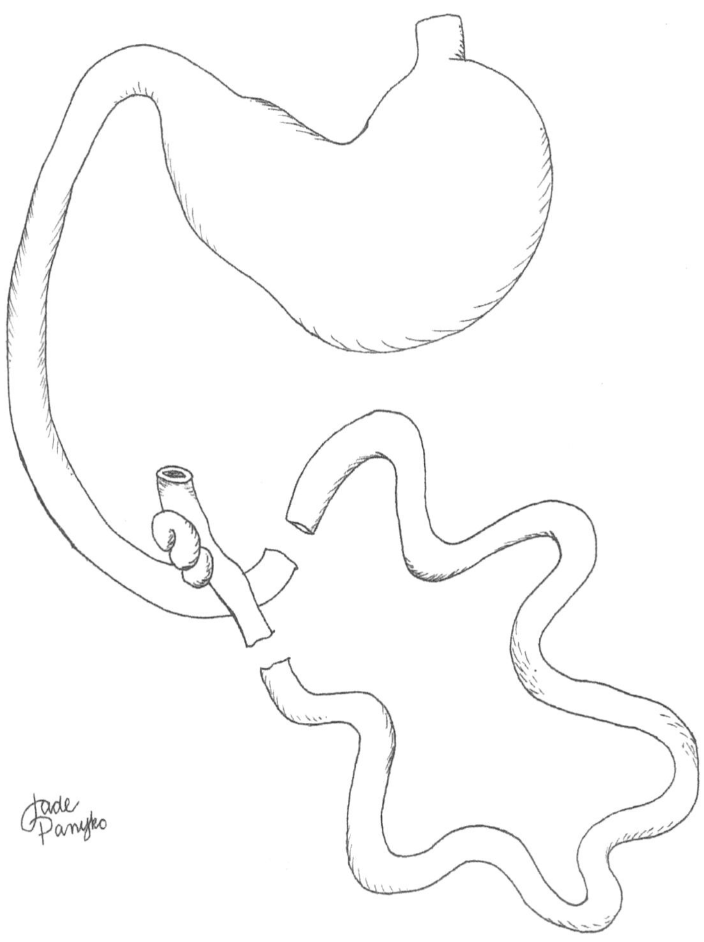

Their Small Intestine

- The first part of the small intestine, called the duodenum, receives bile from the liver and gallbladder that emulsifies fat and bicarbonate from the pancreas to neutralize the acidity of the stomach.
- The small intestine in dogs, like most carnivores, has a low acidity. Plus, it is short and smooth with short transit times through the intestinal tract.
- The small intestine has a small amount of microbes or intestinal flora. The total length of the small intestine of a dog is 7-10 feet. This is much shorter compared that to the 21 feet of a human and over a 130 feet of a cow.
- There is minimal ability of a dog to receive energy from carbohydrates from plant based sources, like starches, fiber, or cereal grains. The dog gets its carbohydrates mainly from converting protein or amino acids into glucose in the liver, called gluconeogenesis.

The Colon

- The colon length in a dog is about 2 feet. The human colon is 5 to 6 feet, which is about the same length of a cow. Though this is still a difference, the small intestine length is the main difference between the carnivore, omnivore and herbivore.
- Because dog are carnivores, if they were kept in the zoo, they would get what most carnivores get – meat and bones. Most commercial dog food, however, is 25 % protein, and the rest is complex and simple carbohydrates consistent with what a herbivore would eat, which is exactly opposite of the biological diet and nutritional requirements for good dog health.

- Normal transit time for a dog eating meat and bones is 4 to 6 hours. The transit time for non-carnivore diets can increase, causing diarrhea or constipation. Most dogs' bowel movements normalize with a carnivore diet proportioned appropriately for dog size, metabolic rate, and level of physical activity of the dog. Keeping dogs hydrated with plenty of water, blocking stress, and providing mostly protein-based diets will usually do the trick.

Their Intestines

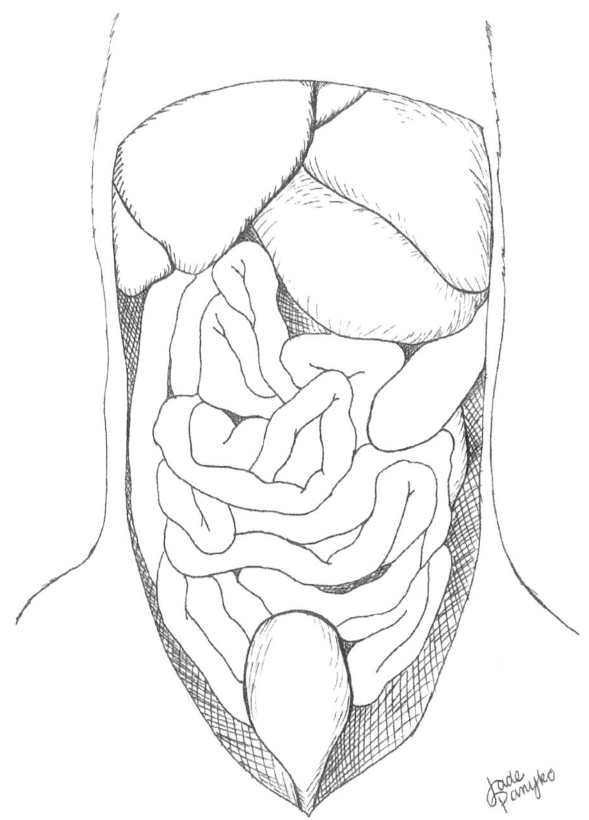

The Endocrine Organs

The Adrenal Gland

- Dogs' adrenal glands are located on top of the kidneys, and they are comprised of two parts: the cortex and the medulla.
- The adrenal gland in dogs is used as a backup to create hormones (testosterone, estrogen, etc.) in the event that a dog is spayed or neutered.
- The adrenal gland is also a backup for other hormone synthesis.
    - Cholesterol can become progesterone. The produced progesterone can then become aldosterone, cortisol or androstenedione.
    - Pregnenolone can become DHEA (Dehydroepiandrosterone). This DHEA can then become androstenedione. Androstenedione can become testosterone, which can then become either DHT (Dihydrotestosterone) or estrogen.
- The adrenal gland can become overstimulated. This can lead to:
    - Increased aldosterone, which leads to hypertension.
    - Increased cortisol, which damages the brain and body.
    - Decreased progesterone.
    - Decreased thyroid, or thyroid function, which causes a hypothyroid condition.

The Endocrine Organs

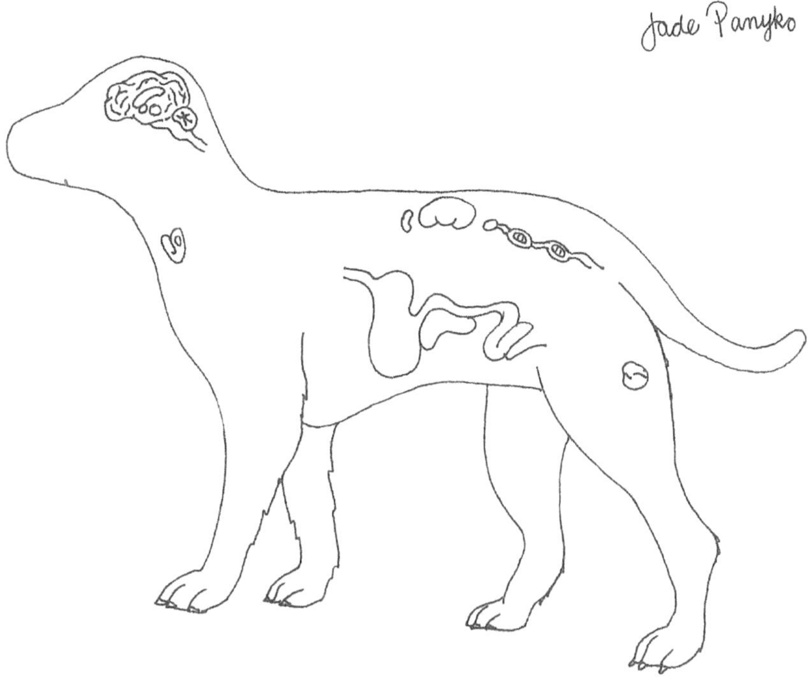

XIV. Dogs: Their Reproduction and Controlling It

Female Anatomy

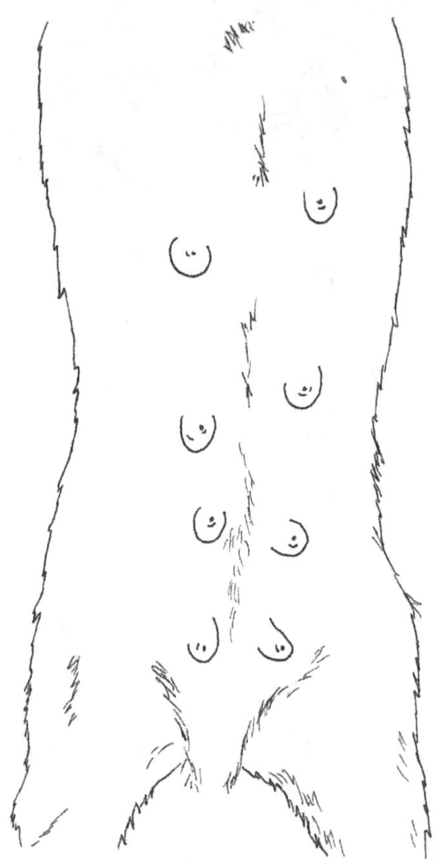

Male Anatomy

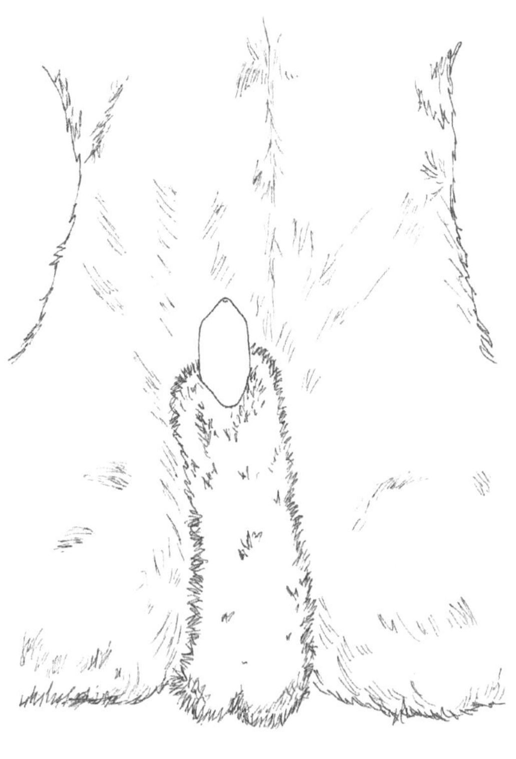

Jade Panyko

Why It's Done

- ➢ Population control is one of the main reasons. There are 6.5 million animals in animal shelters and only 3.2 million find a home annually.
- ➢ Some pet owners do this in order control their dog's behavior. For example, they want their male dog to be less aggressive.

- However, the testosterone for dogs helps with muscle health, especially in growing dogs.
- Cortisol in the short term has both anti-inflammatory properties (decreases muscle and joint pain) and is needed for gluconeogenesis (making glucose), which is especially necessary during fight or flight sympathetic action responses of the dog. Long-term exposure to cortisol is detrimental to the mobility of the dog, as the spine, bones, muscles, and joints are adversely affected. Moreover, cortisol exposure decreases the normal digestive function of the dog that will ultimately produce less energy for the dog and over the long term weaken the dog's immune system.

Spaying Female Dogs

- This procedure removes both ovaries or removes the ovaries and the uterus.
- This is typically performed before the first heat cycle, which takes place in female dogs between 5 and 10 months. Usually, this is done when the dog is 4 to 6 months old.
- Some claim that this procedure reduces the risk of breast cancer, but this has been challenged and is a not universally agreed upon, as breast cancer in dogs has more to do with the balance of estrogen and progesterone as opposed to just removal or decrease of estrogen.
- Because this can have significant consequences, some already discussed in this book, a better method is to wait until a dog reaches a more mature age or tie the tubes of the female-rather than removing her reproductive organs.
- Female dogs can undergo a sterilization procedure that removes the uterus and one ovary but leaves one ovary intact, which will not compromise the sterilization and will provide

favorable benefits for the health of the dog, including brain, heart, and bone health for starters.

Neutering: Male Dogs

- This procedure removes the male's testes.
- This is typically performed when the dog is between 4 and 6 months.
- Neutering obviously eliminates the risk of testicular cancer in the male dog, as the testes are gone; however, there is concern of an increased risk in prostate cancer due to increase in estrogen, which means the hormones are not balanced with testosterone.
- Because of the significant consequences, some already discussed in this book, a better method is to wait until the dog is more mature in age and perform a vasectomy. [60] Doing this will allow for the dog to preserve testosterone for muscle development and health.

The Issues

- As stated above, there are issues with performing these procedures.
- The adrenal gland is forced to work overtime as a hormone production center, creating estrogen and testosterone that was once made in the reproductive organs.
- There are high levels of ACTH (adrenocorticotropic hormone) in a dog's adrenal glands, which stimulates and increases the secretion of cortisol. "The constant effort of the brain to tell the adrenal gland it needs sex hormones creates

---

60. Digesting Bones, Gastric Acidity, Salmonella in Dogs and Cats." Vets All Natural, October 19, 2018. https://vetsallnatural.com.au/digesting-bones-gastric-acidity-salmonella-dogs-cats/?s=.

a continuous signal to inadvertently produce cortisol, which long term is bad for the dog's brain and body."[61]

- Furthermore, since the adrenal gland and thyroid gland work opposite of each other as the adrenal gland is working harder, the thyroid gland is under active or hypothyroid. In effect, both the adrenal and thyroid gland are working against the health of the body.

A Better Solution

- At 4 to 6 months of age of a dog needs both some testosterone and some estrogen, with males needing more testosterone and females needing more estrogen.
- The brain and heart need estrogen and testosterone, as do the muscles, joints, and bones. The adrenal gland is the back-up endocrine organ in the absence of reproductive organs.
- Performing a vasectomy and tying a dog's tubes or leaving an ovary allows the dog's body to generate the hormones needed, while negating long-term effects of an overactive adrenal gland and subsequently underactive thyroid gland.

61. "Explore Hormones,Observation, Treatment Details from Idea Clinics." Idea Clinics, 2020. https://www.ideaclinics.com/hormones-section/.

XV. Dogs: Their Diet

- Dogs are scavengers and will eat anything, but they are obligate carnivores. They need meat and bones.
- Dogs have a relatively short gastrointestinal tract. It is the length primarily of the small intestine that reflects and should determine the type of diet consumed. As a general guide: A dog or any other carnivore has a small intestine that is 7 to 10 feet; people or other omnivores have a small intestine around 21-22 feet, and cows or other herbivores have a small intestine around 120 -130 feet long. Herbivores have a small intestine that is nearly 20 times their body length.
- Dogs gastrointestinal tract is good for easily and quickly digesting raw meat, but plants and vegetables can take significantly longer and should be considerably restricted.
- "Fresh meat can be digested and processed in the carnivores body in as little as 4-6 hours, whereas plant and vegetable material in a herbivore's gut can take 3-5 days to be processed"
- Dogs should drink plenty of water, as the metabolism of protein, which should be the main food source, requires plenty of water.
- Dogs do not sweat, so maintaining the dog's body temperature both in cold and hot weather requires access to a plentiful supply of water. In hot weather the dog pants to keep cool again requiring plenty of water.

XVI. Dogs: The Dog "Feed" Problem

- We feed dogs like they are cows. Said another way, we are feeding our dog as if it was an herbivore instead of acknowledging what it actually is, an obligate or strict carnivore.
- Metabolizing food is the biggest health problem, digestively, that dogs face.
- Veterinarians are not trained in nutrition education for animals, which needs to change.
- What we feed our dogs can contribute to the cause, spread, and symptoms of cancer, diabetes, obesity, allergies, yeast infections, joint pain and issues, and ear problems.
- High starch, highly processed foods or non- diverse foods for prolonged period of time can lead to cancer, poor diet, and chronic inflammation.
- Processed commercial and grain- based diets damage mitochondria, as a low energy state is created. Dogs get their energy from glucose and ketones (fat breakdown). The glucose is derived from protein or amino acids and produced in the liver by a process called gluconeogenesis. When the dog is not eating, the fat can be broken down in the liver as ketones, giving dogs an alternative energy source.
- The generation of cancer or tumors in dogs is a low energy production problem, while the spread of cancer is generally an impaired immune system.
- In 1970, 1 in every 10 dogs developed cancer; now, it is 1 in 2 dogs, and this can be attributed to a mismatch of the biological nutrition regarding what a dog needs versus what is given. Either way the brain and body of the dog is not getting what is needed for optimal dog health and over time there are consequences.

- Processed foods also destroy a dog's micro biome; however the dog's micro biome, especially in the small intestine, is much more restricted than in omnivores and herbivores.
- Dogs can suffer from gastrointestinal problems due to preservatives and artificial ingredients in their food, which is a poor substitute for quality protein, which is mainly what the dog really needs.
- "What we see with the advent of processed pet foods, is a significant change in the general nature of ingredients in the diet. It is a simple commercial fact that meat protein is the most expensive component in any pet food, and as a result, there is always commercial pressure to keep meat protein levels to a minimum, thereby keeping costs down of the end product (and / or maximizing profits). Modern processed pet foods have adapted to these financial constraints firstly by significantly increasing the carbohydrate component of dog foods"[62]
- Processed pet foods also use plant-based protein, again due to the fact that they are cheaper, and this in turn adversely impacts the digestion and integrity of the gastrointestinal tract of the dog.[63]
- The processed food diets often given to dogs, with high carbohydrates and plant-based proteins, decrease the acidity level in the stomach, which can lead to several issues; with regard to proper digestion, everything starts with getting the stomach to work optimally as there is a cascade of events that follow, none of which are good.
- There are no food regulations or laws for pet food, so anything can be in the food because the dog food is not even termed food, it is classified as feed. Dog food is regulated not by the FDA but by the Department of Agriculture.

62. "Digesting Bones, Gastric Acidity, Salmonella in Dogs and Cats." Vets All Natural, October 19, 2018. https://vetsallnatural.com.au/digesting-bones-gastric-acidity-salmonella-dogs-cats/?s=.
63. Ibid.

- There are many harmful bacteria in dry dog food (kibble). These can include listeria, e. Coli, and Salmonella.
- Processed dog food mainly consists of carbohydrates that leads to inflammation in dogs.
- GMO's are very toxic to pets' digestive systems and their immune systems.

Carbohydrates and Grain Based Food

- Grain based food is dirt cheap.
- Dry kibble is baked, irradiated, extruded, and full of carbohydrates, none of which is good for dogs. Dogs are not cows. Dogs are carnivores, and cows are herbivores. If you are confused, the dog barks, "Woof," and the cow says, "Moo!"
- Processed dog food is around 28% protein, 8- 20 % fat, and 30 -50% carbohydrates, though dog food companies do not have to list carbohydrates on their ingredients and in fact are prohibited from doing so. The dog's gastrointestinal tract is not designed to process carbohydrates, and this diet is not consistent with good gastrointestinal health in dogs.
- There are no carbohydrates listed on the dog food labels, but the carbohydrate percentage can be determined by adding the protein, fat, ash, water, then taking 100 and subtracting the calculated number to determine the carbohydrate content.
- Carbohydrates include sugars and starches.
- Naturally, dogs in the wild would not have access to carbohydrates. Only about 5-7% of their diet would consist of carbohydrates, meaning their bodies are not designed for the >50% carbohydrate diet dog food provides.

- The pet food industry is essentially a cereal food industry, meaning it's about less healthy, cheaper options for pets. Again, grain based food is cheap.
- Carbohydrate diets lead to diseases and premature death in dogs due to metabolic consequences with decreased energy production and compromised immune health.
- Starch and carbohydrate dog diets significantly decrease a dog's lifespan. A dog that can live to be 14 could die much earlier, say at the age of 7, or if the dog lives longer, the quality of life could be of a lesser quality and less comfortable.

Grain Free Foods

- Grain free foods are extremely expensive; they can cost $100 per bag. Grain free means there is no soy, corn, oats, or wheat.
- When a bag says "grain free," it is still an indication that something could be harmful in the food for a dog's diet.
- Foods that claim to be grain free can still have high levels of sugar. Furthermore, manufactures do not have to write sugar or carbohydrates on the bag. If a bag contains the words rice, corn, lentils, peas, chickpeas, or potatoes, those are other words for high in sugar and starch, even though they are not technically grains.
- Carnivores, such as dogs, are not supposed to eat a lot of starch. The gastrointestinal tract of dogs is designed for protein, but it is never too late to make the switch.

How Veterinarians Contribute to the Problem

- Veterinarians are not trained in nutrition education for animals, which needs to change.

- Vet school is taught in part or at least controlled in part by veterinary pet food companies.
- Veterinarian ignorance on nutrition can lead to frustration.
- Very rarely is a dog's nutrition treated as a crisis by vets, so it goes undiscussed or overlooked, as the consequences are generally not acute problems but rather are chronic or long term problems that are created and are easier to dismiss.
- Misinformation and a lack of knowledge is why veterinarians do not believe in raw diets, which are actually good for dogs.
- Veterinarians are not looking to solve and are not discussing the issues with the commercial pet food industry.

XVII. Solving the Dog "Feed" Problem

- The number one change that can be done to improve dog health is changing their diet.
- Nutrition can be used both as a preventative measure and a treatment.
- Dog nutrition should mimic their ancestry. Dogs are obligate carnivores, who have evolved to eat meat.
- The best thing to do is feed a dog one meal a day, primarily raw meat with the bone
- Providing the appropriate biological nutrition (meat and bones as protein) for the dog is what carnivores require, which is the key to longevity in dogs.

Evidence Based Nutrition

- The studies have already been done on wild animals, like wolves who eat meat and bones as carnivores. These studies predate agriculture and pet feed manufacturing.
- Studies show increased sugar increases inflammation.
- Studies show high carbohydrates alter the pH in dogs, making it harder to break down protein. If your dog has received long-term high carbohydrate pet food, the acidity of the stomach will take weeks to develop as the daily protein diet is re-introduced.
- Studies show an important diet is a fresh meat diet with a few tweaks.

Alternative Energy Sources

- Raw Unprocessed Food Diet
    - Dogs' ancestors have eaten this diet for centuries, and their bodies are designed for it.
    - Once a day feed a dog grass fed meat, healthy fat, and some key vitamins and minerals.

- Cooked fats are a pro-inflammatory, but raw fats are not. Therefore, buy raw meat in bulk and freeze it, but do not cook the fat.
- This type of diet contains natural enzymes to aid in digestion, digestion repair, and lower inflammation.
- This diet can consist of any raw meat: muscle, bone, cartilage, and organ meat.
- Things like raw meats and unpasteurized milk leads to healthier digestive health in dogs; this is in contrast to diets with pasteurized milk and cooked meat, which leads to degenerative diseases.
- This type of diet protects dogs from bacterial contamination and food poisoning.
- Furthermore, this will make it easier for dogs to consume and chew on bones.
- "It is a fact that dogs that eat processed foods are even more likely to shed salmonella bacteria than are dogs that eat raw food."[64]
- "The low PH also is highly effective at killing bacteria, particularly potentially pathogenic bacteria like Salmonella, Clostridia, Campylobacter and E Coli. In fact, natural 'wild' diets of dogs have evolved a more favorable gastric environment that favors the breakdown of raw meats, raw bones, and a pH that kills potentially harmful bacteria – consistent with the requirements of carnivores, and in particular, the scavenging nature of dogs."[65]
- Provide dogs fresh chicken, beef, and turkey with their nutrients and give them patties (liver) once a week.

64. Ibid.
65. Ibid.

- Most problems reported when dogs change abruptly to a raw diet occur as a result of their previous processed food diet , which can be mitigated by transitioning in stages rather than all at once.
- With dogs who have eaten processed dog food, their pH levels are higher (more alkaline) and their digestion has slowed down. This means that changing to this diet may take time.
- "If you intend to feed meat or a raw food diet, you must make this change gradually over 7-10 days...dogs can handle it if it is introduced gradually, and the gastric acidity is allowed to normalize," but they may vomit if you start the process too quickly.[66]
- Furthermore, "with the altered pH, raw bones and material is not softened and broken down effectively (digestive enzymes lose function), and this can result in obstruction... These dogs already have a less acidic stomach, which is not able to soften and breakdown raw bone material, nor is the stomach PH able to cope with a load of bacteria. The result can be a sudden 'rejection' of the bone or meat, in the form of vomiting, or it can take the form of a bout of acute gastroenteritis, from an overgrowth of bacteria, or it may result in a bone obstruction in the stomach"[67]
- It is not just raw meats that can help dogs, but key minerals and vitamins can be added to aid in their health as well. To keep the body functioning optimally, there must be the proper configuration of proteins and specific minerals and vitamins.

- Ketogenic Diet:
  - By definition, the correct diet for a dog is a carnivore diet consisting of meat and bones, which already is a ketogenic

66. Ibid.
67. Ibid.

diet due to the fact that in this diet carbohydrates are not only restricted, they are absent.

- Dogs obtain glucose when needed by converting protein or amino acids in the liver by a process called gluconeogenesis
- Dogs like Huskies or sled dogs burn a lot of calories and will need more fat in their diet as under these high energy burning conditions consuming more calories is of paramount importance and the composition of the calories is a secondary issue.

- Intermittent Fasting
  - Dogs should intermittently fast a couple times a week. If they normally eat twice a day, just change to once a day meals.
  - Many dogs do this naturally.
  - Fasting is an anti-angiogenic and anti-inflammatory, and it produces anti-cancer cells. The same applies to people: if you want to live longer, eat less.
  - This type of diet slows down cancer and prevents it in dogs who are not already diagnosed.
- Supplements to a Dog's Diet:
  - Minerals: Magnesium, Potassium, and Calcium (if not adding bones to the meat)
  - Vitamin D3/K2
  - Key amino acids: glutamine, tyrosine, and tryptophan
  - Anti-inflammatory: turmeric and omega 3
  - Antioxidants: glutathione and alpha lipoic acid
  - Iodine and zinc
  - B-vitamins for brain, liver, and energy metabolism

XVIII. Dogs: Their Facial Expressions and Posture

- Dogs use their facial expressions and posture, more than barking, to communicate. This communication can express their mood and health.[68]
- Dogs are masters at communication with both facial expression and body posturing, meaning they can say little, if anything, at all.
- Even small movements, like head tilts and facial expressions, are important for dog communication.

Four Common Facial Expressions

Head Tilting

- This occurs when a dogs turns its head to one side or moves his head from side to side.
- This conveys curiosity, but it also means the dog is relaxed.[69]
- When a dog does this, it is telling you that it is "all ears" and is fully focused on you at that moment.

Flattening Ears

- The dog pulls or presses their ears tight to the head, flattening them.
- This can convey either fear or aggression.
    - If a dog is fearful, its forehead will be smooth, and it will be in a cowering position. [70]

---

68. Stephens, Jack. "4 Dog Facial Expressions and What They Mean." Pet Insurance Blog - Pets Best Insurance, September 6, 2019. https://www.petsbest.com/blog/4-dog-facial-expressions/?CI=5000002&spJobID=1282884924&spMailingID=55376158&spReportId=MTI4Mjg4NDkyNAS2&spUserID=MTcyMDc4MzM1MDI4S0&utm_campaign=Newsletter&utm_medium=email&utm_source=PHS
69. Ibid.
70. Ibid.

- If a dog is aggressive, the forehead will be tense and wrinkled, and it may be snarling.[71]

Eyebrow Raising

- This occurs when a dog lifts one or both eyebrows. It gives them the appearance of having a wide-eyed look.
- This means the dogs may be surprised, astonished, or uncertain.
- This mostly takes place when they receive a treat or reward when they were not expecting it.

Head Bowing

- This stance happens when a dog lowers its head or is flat on the ground as the eyes look up in a non-threatening manner.
- This means that the dog may be unsure, shy, or anxious about the situation or is choosing to be submissive.
    - A dog may be unsure when they are meeting a new person or another dog.
    - A dog may submissive to avoid a fight.

71. Ibid.

XIX. Dogs: Their Tails

- Dogs also use their tails as a method of communicating several things, including their mood and mindset. "Without the ability to speak past barks, tail positioning and motion allows dogs (with tails) to make various emotions known."[72]

- People should be cautious when approaching a new dog and consider their body posture, tail wags, and tail position before attempting to pet the dog.

Tail Wagging

- Many people instantly think of tail wagging when discussing dogs' tails, and while it is a common belief that tail wagging means the dog is happy, that is not always the case.

- Tail wagging is an indicator of a dog's right and left-brain relationships.

Wagging to the Right

- A tail wag to the right means a dog is happy.
- " A right wag tail position indicates happiness and playfulness as the left brain controls the right side of the body as well as energy and engagement responses."[73]

Wagging to the Left

- A wagging to the left is an indicator that a dog is fearful.
- "As opposed to a left wag tail position indicates insecurity and restlessness; the right brain hemisphere controls the

---

72. Erus, Nola. "Dog Tail Positions and What They Mean." BarkleyAndPaws, n.d. https://www.barkleyandpaws.com/dogs/health/dog-tail-positions-and-what-they-mean.
73. Ibid.

body's left side of the dogs body including the direction of the tail wagging."[74]

Wagging Low

➢ A low tail wag shows nervousness.

Wagging Rapidly

➢ A rapid tail wag, when coupled with tense muscle, signals aggression.

Tail Positions

➤ Outside of wagging movement, there are three common tail positions for dogs: up high, horizontal to the ground, and down/between their hind legs. It is important to know what each of them mean.[75]

Up High

➢ This indicates that the dog feels confident, powerful, and secure; essentially, this dog sees themselves as a dominant alpha.

➢ "Confidence, however, comes with a certain coolness. Self-assured, the dominant, tail up dog communicates power and control via body language, and this is often sufficient for delivery clear 'Don't cross me' messages to other dogs. With his tail high, a dog releases much more of his signature scent from his anal gland, and this acts as an announcement, too."[76]

74. Ibid.
75. Ibid.
76. Ibid.

Horizontal to the Ground

- This is a more neutral tail position, and a dog displaying this may be more curious than anything.
- "Their unrelaxed but non-assertive position indicates curiosity rather than reactionary assertiveness or relinquishment of control. Perhaps you have noticed your own dog coming closer when you have someone new or an unusual item with you. Set on go for exploration, he puts his tail out in the same way he might perk his ears inquisitively."[77]

Down/Between Hind Legs

- A dog presenting its tail between his hind legs is showing submissive behavior.
- "With his tail in the down/between hind legs position, a dog communicates an understanding of another's dominant position and his submissive one…A tucked tail will hinder release of a dog's signature scent, and in this way the dog may expect to go unnoticed by other dogs."[78]

---

77. Ibid.
78. Ibid.

XX. Dogs: Their Emotions

- Dogs can experience the basic emotions of happiness, sadness, and fear.
- Dogs can also experience more complex emotions, such as jealousy; however, they display it differently than humans.
- Dogs are very empathic.
- "A dog can detect fear or anxiety and either protect or take an offensive position depending on the circumstance. Additionally, if the owner is sad or ill the dog can empathize and provide a comforting position and demeanor."[79]

Jealousy in Dogs

- Dogs typically become jealous when someone or another dog receives a reward when they received nothing.
- Signs of their jealousy include displaying signs of agitation, avoiding contact with the human or dog, and scratching frequently.[80]
- "An interesting aspect of their feeling of jealousy is in the lack of importance of what's being offered as a reward. If one dog is being given something great as a treat such as a piece of steak while another is given something like a small dog biscuit, the signs of jealousy are not present. They only care that they get rewarded, not what the reward is."[81]

---

79. "Dog Psychology – 10 Facts on How Your Dog's Mind Works." The Fabulous Dog Bed Company, May 17, 2018. https://www.thefabulousdogbedcompany.co.uk/blog/read_184273/dog-psychology-10-facts-on-how-your-dogs-mind-works.html.
80. Ibid.
81. Ibid.

Guilt in Dogs

- Dogs, contrary to popular opinion, do not experience guilt. Instead they experience sadness because their owner is mad or because they were caught.
- For example, when a person walks into a room and sees that the dog has destroyed something, the dogs typically sits there with a sad expression. However, they are not sad they did it; "when a dog sees the look of disapproval on their owner's face or hears anger and disappointment in their voice, they react negatively, with expressions of sadness."[82]
- The above fact also means that dogs don't frame other dogs intentionally to make them feel guilty. Dogs react to their owner's tone of voice not the deed itself.

Revenge in Dogs

- Dogs do not possess the brain capacity required for them to think ahead and commit premeditated revenge. Instead, they immediately react.
- Dogs do not actively seek revenge or have a vengeful streak, though many times dog owners feel this is the case.
- For example, a dog might go to the bathroom on the carpet when their owners leave, or they tear up the carpet, a pillow, or the couch.
- This behavior can be explained for other reasons. "The dog could have gone to the bathroom on the carpet because it was stressed out from being home alone all day or having a drastic change in routine (or) ...the dog could have been frustrated due to pent up energy from not

82. Ibid.

being played with and released the energy through tearing something up."[83]

- "The bad acts should be addressed through proper methods such as stress management and alternative play time not punishment."[84]

83. Ibid.
84. Ibid.

XXI. Dogs: Their Perception of Time

- Dogs do not truly have the ability to perceive time as they cannot create and store long-term memories. "Humans can consciously and willfully think back to specific memories and anticipate and plan for the future events, but dogs cannot think or plan in the future."[85]
- Though they do not understand the concept of time, dogs do have an "internal clock" that reminds them when food is likely to be served or owners are likely to return from work. This is purely a biological reaction to a specific time of day, however, and has nothing to do with memorizing time.
- Dogs have a working short-term memory, but it fades very quickly.
- The Difference: Humans understand time in two ways.
  - We remember events as a sequence.
  - We can anticipate the future- things that will happen or things that we will need.

---

85. "How Long Do You Leave Your Dog?" ArabianLines.Com Forum, August 21, 2010. http://arabianlines.com/forum1/topic_new.asp?TOPIC_ID=42190&whichpage=2.

XXII. Dogs: Their Sleep and Sleep Patterns

- "Dogs share similar sleep patterns as humans, and their brain activity while sleeping also resembles that of a human brain when asleep." [86]
- Dogs most likely can dream, similar to the way a person does, and "the most common dreams are happy and involve activities such as playing, chasing an animal, or simply running around."[87]
- A dog's sleep patterns are biologically opposite the human sleep cycle, meaning the dog normally should sleep during the day and be active at night. This stems from their biological need to hunt for food, but just as people can change their sleep patterns (working the night shift) domesticated dogs change their sleep cycles.
- Dogs do produce melatonin, as humans do. However, in people melatonin increases as it gets dark out and increases a person's ability to sleep. Since wolves hunt at night, if melatonin were truly only mediated by darkness to increase levels, the wolves would sleep during darkness and miss out on hunting for food; clearly, this is not the case.
- Melatonin is not as important in mammals for day/night cycle. Besides light, temperature also regulates melatonin with colder temperatures increasing melatonin and warmer temperatures decreasing melatonin, which better explains how wolves regulate their melatonin and have a different sleepy cycle than that of humans (hunting during the darkness and sleeping during the light).

---

86. "Dog Psychology – 10 Facts on How Your Dog's Mind Works." The Fabulous Dog Bed Company, May 17, 2018. https://www.thefabulousdogbedcompany.co.uk/blog/read_184273/dog-psychology-10-facts-on-how-your-dogs-mind-works.html.
87. Ibid.

- Melatonin is produced from serotonin and norepinephrine; therefore, tryptophan and tyrosine, plus cofactors, can facilitate sleep. These are more likely to be available on a carnivore's diet of protein than an omnivore's diet.

Dogs: Their Training

- "If dogs don't receive some form of discipline through effective and consistent training and their owners taking a dominant stance, they can easily become unhappy (and) confused in what is and is not acceptable behave."[88]
- Training is also important for them to feel accepted and happy. "Dogs need a healthy balance of affection, attention, and discipline in order to feel secure, safe, happy, and like a true part of the family."[89]
- Dogs can be trained best when they have an older, already trained dog with them. They can see the desired behavior and learn how to react and follow commands.
- "Puppies commonly model their behavior from older dogs in their household. If the older dog is trained well and behaves, the puppy can adopt the behavior of the dog quite quickly."
- Furthermore, "when the older dog is given a command, performs it and gets a treat, the puppy may be able to more easily understand what this command means and what to do when it is given through a form of mimicry "[90]

88. Ibid.
89. Ibid.
90. Ibid.

XXIII. Dogs: What Can Go Wrong

- Dogs, like humans, can experience an entire host of problems, including obesity, arthritis, organ degeneration, autoimmune diseases, allergies, immune dysfunction and metabolic diseases, and adrenal and thyroid issues.
- Dogs can develop the same chronic diseases and cancer as humans.
- Most powerful interventions never get studied because there is no monetary incentive to do so.

Mitochondria

- Mitochondrial dense tissues are in the dog's brain, heart, kidney, and liver. Muscles are also full of mitochondria.
- Are we misunderstanding the nature of the biology of disease in dogs? There needs to be more of a focus on the mitochondria and energy production of the cells in the brain and body of dogs, which is best supported by giving the dog the correct nutrition and diet.
- Mitochondria have their own DNA with weaker repair mechanisms.
- Mitochondria are fueled by glucose and oxygen , but they can also be fueled by ketones as a reserve fuel during fasting.
- Dogs can get chronic diseases and cancer from damaged and/or decreased mitochondria. Cells need energy or ATP to function. Low energy creates oxidative stress and free radicals creating cell damage with subsequent inflammation.
- Mitochondria senses their local environment:
    - Cell (nucleus) senses low energy or energy crisis from decreased energy production by the mitochondria.
    - Cancer genes (oncogenes) know there is basically 2 possible courses of action either prepare the cell for

apoptosis or cell death or create conditions that change the mitochondria to shift the energy source from aerobic to anaerobic metabolism as the cells rapidly divide as a tumor or cancer.

- Since not all cells can divide (for example: brain (neurons), heart, and skeletal muscle cells cannot divide), the only choice when mitochondria produce low energy is apoptosis or cell death. However, glial cells in the brain can divide as brain cancer, unlike neurons that would die and manifest as brain atrophy.

Diseases

Rabies

➢ Rabies is caused by a virus that manifests 1 to 2 months after infected.

➢ The dog may exhibit wanting to be left alone and anxious behaviors, followed by uncharacteristic aggressive behavior.

➢ A dog with rabies is very sensitive to noise, and advanced rabies can cause paralysis, especially of the head and neck. The mouth can remain open from paralyzed muscles, and there is difficulty swallowing as saliva drips from the dog's open mouth.

➢ The best prevention for a dog developing rabies is vaccination.

Parvovirus

➢ This is a virus that affects dogs, causing gastrointestinal changes including vomiting and bloody diarrhea from inflammation of the intestinal tract with possible problems with dehydration and electrolyte abnormalities.

➢ The dog may stop eating until the condition improves.

- The inflammation of the intestinal tract can create an immune problem, putting the dog at risk for secondary infection.
- A protein diet is important for dogs to mitigate risk of infection.
- Supportive care is generally what is needed for favorable outcomes.

Distemper

- All dogs are at risk of infection from distemper virus, but it generally affects puppies under 6 months.
- The disease affects the respiratory and gastrointestinal systems and later the central nervous system.
- Respiratory symptoms include sneeze, cough, or thick mucus affecting the nose as frequent discharge. Worsening systems can involve the lungs and labored breathing. Mucus discharge from eyes and nose suggests distemper, especially if the dog is not vaccinated.
- High fever and poor appetite mean dehydration can quickly develop. Dehydration can worsen if vomiting or diarrhea become symptoms that the dog has.
- The pads of the dog's feet can also become sensitive.
- Teeth development, including enamel deposition, can be interrupted.
- Seizures can be a late sign of distemper.
- Dogs infected with distemper virus are extremely ill and will need consultation with your veterinarian. Acute intervention may involve intravenous fluid, electrolyte replacement, and nutritional support that provides protein and glucose.

Hypothyroidism

- Hypothyroidism is a condition that affects a dog's metabolism because the thyroid hormone that controls metabolism is not being produced as it should be. A normal thyroid function is consistent with improved energy metabolism and improved longevity and dog health.
- The high cholesterol stemming from hypothyroidism is also linked to the adrenal gland in dogs that have been spayed or neutered.
- The main cause of an underactive thyroid in dogs is due to an overactive adrenal gland. Dogs that have been spayed or neutered have an over stimulated adrenal gland trying to producing hormones, such as estrogen and testosterone, that were lowered by removing either the ovaries or testes at the time of a sterilization procedure.
- Low thyroid levels in a dog can change their overall brain structure and its function, especially during the brain development of the dog.
- Fatigue is a common symptom of hypothyroidism. "Many dogs with the condition…are unable to go about their day as usual. The fatigue occurs regardless of how much sleep a dog gets or how many daytime naps they take."[91]
- Another symptom of hypothyroidism is weight gain, as the dog has a low level of thyroid hormones, which are used to regulate body weight, intake of food, and metabolism.[92]
- A third symptom of hypothyroidism is sore muscle and joints, which can be stiff, swollen, tender, or weak.

---

91. Leonard, Jayne. "Hypothyroidism Symptoms: 12 Signs to Look out For." Medical News Today. MediLexicon International, February 25, 2019. https://www.medicalnewstoday.com/articles/324535.
92. Ibid.

- "There is a link between hypothyroid disorders and arthritis, which is an autoimmune condition that causes painful swelling in the lining of the joints. The low thyroid combined with high cortisol creates gastrointestinal dysfunctions as the sympathetic system is chronically stimulated with the parasympathetic lowered to diminish the rest, digestion, and repair mechanisms of the dog."[93]
- A fourth symptom is changes in a dog's mood and memory.
- "It is common for dogs with untreated hypothyroidism to experience apathy, or general lack of interest or feelings of indifference, impaired memory function, less attentiveness and concentration, and lower mood or even anxiety."[94]
- Dogs with hypothyroidism can also feel cold. "Hypothyroidism can slow down metabolism, which can lead to a drop in core body temperature."[95]
- "An underactive thyroid can cause problems with movement through the gut and the activity of the stomach, small intestine, and colon."[96] One example, of this would be the dog experiencing constipation.
- "The consequences for a dog with constipation can include: hard stools, difficulty passing stool, or a feeling of being unable to empty the rectum fully."[97]
- A seventh symptom for dogs with hypothyroidism is high cholesterol as the high cholesterol levels are the dog's response to inflammation. With inflammation comes an increase in cholesterol. .

---

93. Ibid.
94. Ibid.
95. Ibid.
96. Ibid.
97. Ibid.

- “Thyroid hormones play a vital role in removing excess cholesterol from the body via the liver. Low thyroid levels mean that the liver struggles to carry out this function and blood cholesterol levels increase.”[98]
- Dogs with hypothyroidism may also develop a slower heart rate, a condition called bradycardia. “Bradycardia can cause weakness, dizziness, and breathing problems. Without treatment, this heart condition may result in serious complications, such as high or low blood pressure or heart failure.[99]
- However, the heart can be affected in other ways by this condition, such as blood pressure changes, varied heart rhythms, or hardened/less elastic arteries.[100]
- A ninth hypothyroidism symptom is hair loss for dogs because the hormones produced by the thyroid regulate hair growth.
- “Dogs with more severe thyroid problems are more prone to developing alopecia, which is an autoimmune condition that cause hair to fall out in patches.”[101]
- Dry skin and weak hair or nails can be yet another indicator that a dog has hypothyroidism.
- Dry, scaly skin and a constant itching may develop in dogs with this condition. This is due to the fact the thyroid hormones affect skin and fur.[102]
- An eleventh sign of hypothyroidism in dogs is goiters.

98. Ibid.
99. Ibid.
100. Ibid.
101. Ibid.
102. Ibid.

- "Enlargement of the thyroid gland that appears as swelling at the base of the neck. Other goiter symptoms include problems swallowing and breathing. Many thyroid problems can result in a goiter, which may manifest as a thyroiditis, which is an autoimmune condition that damages the thyroid gland, stopping it producing enough hormones."[103]
- All the symptoms listed above, even changed brain function, can be reversed when treated.
- A way to prevent hypothyroidism to not spay and neuter dogs, but instead to leave at least one ovary in females and perform a vasectomy in males. This is in addition to giving the dog a protein diet (Tyrosine) that contains a few minerals (iodine) and B-vitamins.

Cancer

- Cancer is very common among dogs. However, there is not much cancer in the wild.
- Dogs have the highest cancer rate of any animal.
- Cancer is essentially a cell growth that is fast dividing and disrupts the normal cell cycle.
- Cancer is a metabolic disease.
- Cancer spread or metastasis occurs in an impaired immune system.
- All types of cancer are seen in dogs, suggesting that there is an abnormal underlying metabolic process that has gone wrong.
- Over 80% of cancer research is non-reproducible or not done on what matters. The quality of research is based on the quality of questions being asked. Independent think tanks

103. Ibid.

interested in improving the quality of dog health is a primary goal of Global Health Science Solutions LLC. This company had an interest in promoting animal health in general.

- ➢ The mitochondria and a low energy state effects occurs first because the cell's nucleus is responding to the low energy state in the mitochondria.
- ➢ Insulin is trophic for cancer. Insulin is needed for health, but it needs to be provided intermittently; insulin in the blood all the time is counter productive to good health.

Fleas and Ticks

- ➢ To treat and prevent fleas, don't use over priced products.
- ➢ The dog's sense of smell is very sensitive, be mindful of essential oils that could be irritating or noxious to the dog's sense of smell.
- ➢ Soap and water work well for fleas for your dog. I will leave the best method to implement this to the individual owner and preferences of your dog.

Heartworm

- ➢ Heartworm is a parasitic roundworm that lives in the blood vessels of heart and lungs
- ➢ A blood test by your Veterinarian can confirm if positive for heartworm.
- ➢ It is spread to dogs through mosquito bites and transmitters of heartworm to your dog
- ➢ Heartworm infects the dog's heart and lungs causing lingering dry coughing, respiratory distress or decreased exercise tolerance (fatigue).

- Your veterinarian can provide heartworm pills, other options or considerations include providing Diatomaceous Earth, Coconut oil and garlic are other options that are anti-parasitic that can be mixed with dog food in order to prevent heartworm.

XXIV. Dogs: Taking Care of Them

- Vaccines prevent one disease, but they lower immunity overall in dogs. Therefore, only healthy dogs should be vaccinated.
- No dog under 3 months should receive a vaccine.
- Vaccines should be given in a dog's leg or tail, not the neck.
- Vaccines must be done specific to each dog. Vaccines for dogs are given at the same dose generally, despite wide variations in the size of dogs.
- Vaccine titers could tell if a dog is protected from a disease, obviating the need for yearly vaccinations.
- Dog vaccines are bundled with dog physical exams, and with some 60 million households in the United States owning a dog, the veterinarian dog costs are over $10 billion annually. (All pets in the United States makes up a $100 billion industry.)
- Rabies Vaccine
  - This vaccine is given when a puppy is 6 months old and is usually given at a separate time than the other vaccines
  - Rabies vaccine has mercury as a preservative, so doses must be monitored.
  - A big dog will need one full dose of the rabies vaccine, but a smaller dog will not need the full dose.
  - The rabies vaccine is given every three years, and it should be given anywhere but in the neck.
- Parvovirus, Distemper, and Adenovirus vaccines are usually given together as a combination DP vaccine. A puppy or dog under 12 pounds should only receive a half dose of distemper.
- Bordetella (Kennel Cough) Vaccine can be given at same time as DAP vaccine.

- Leptospirosis Vaccine is usually given to dogs, but the more important vaccines for dogs are Rabies, Distemper and Parvovirus.
- There is a Lyme Disease Vaccine. However, this vaccine does not work. Do not get it for your dog.
- You should only give dogs one vaccine at a time and 3 months apart; however, this is frequently not done as 4-5 vaccines are often given at one time.
- Vaccines can cause issues for dogs, and dogs who become sick as a result of a vaccine can experience degeneration and immune failure.
- There are adjuvant and chemical preservatives in vaccines that can generate an inflammatory response in a dog's immune system.
- The ideal time to vaccinate your dog is every 3 to 6 years; however, there is a range of opinions Some feel an owner just needs immunizations once in the dog's lifetime, but others believe in yearly vaccinations. Still others consider every 6 years as the more best option while there is a 3 year recommendation that serves as a compromise between every one and every 6 years.
- Rather than vaccinating your dog every year, you can measure titers to determine if the vaccine is lasting. If you are unsure if a dog needs a vaccine, you can perform a titer check for circulating antibodies. If the dog titer is positive, then the dog is actively immunized.
- Some dogs are receiving vaccines that are 10 times more potent than necessary. This is because these vaccine have a longer shelf-life; however, less important is the dog's immune response and considerations to the vaccine.

Treating Cancer

- Radiation can play a role in a dog's cancer treatment.
- A change to the dog's biologically correct carnivore diet, meaning a diet consisting mainly of protein, can help a dog fight cancer.
- Surgery for cancer in dogs should be about containment. There should be a get it all or get nothing approach.
- Owners should increase the immune system to stop metastasis. Newer approaches involving chemokine (a type of cytokine or protein messengers) blockade of cell signaling will likely prove more promising in the future regarding stopping the metastasis or the spread of cancer.
- The generation of dog cancer is usually a metabolic or low energy production problem involving the cell's mitochondria, while the spread of cancer is more of an immune problem.

The Veterinary Issue

- Veterinarians are not trained in all the areas they should be, such as nutrition.
- Veterinary offices are treated like a business designed to get pets in the door, give them as many vaccines as possible, prescribe expensive drugs, and sell prescription foods.
- The veterinary industry has become a monopoly to make money- supporting the processed food industry, giving vaccines, etc.
- Banfield bought out over 900 veterinarian hospitals and 250 franchises, as the veterinarian industry has moved from small business toward the monopoly game of big business.

- Over the last 50 years, the diet changes for pets has been the worst in history, and this is a trend that desperately needs to be reversed.
- The American Holistic Veterinary Medical Association is a resource for health and wellness for your dog for comparison recommendations.

Dogs: Health

- Exercise improves the immune system by decreasing stress as dogs need plenty of exercise.
- It is important to exercise any dog as this increases their mitochondria, increases their muscle mass, and lessens their body fat. This can include:
    - Walking
    - Sprinting
    - Swimming in a pool (if overweight)
- It is also important to allow your dog to sleep. Remember they are hardwired to sleep during the day and be awake at night, but their sleep patterns will eventually begin to match their owners.
- Follow the diet and nutritional plan by following a carnivorous or mainly protein diet for your dog.

XXV. Dogs: A Different Path to Dog Health

- Dog health should consist of exercise, the proper diet, supplements, and detoxification.
- Never miss giving your dog rigorous exercise.
- Regarding sterilization procedures for dogs, either performing a vasectomy (for males) or tying the fallopian tubes or leaving an ovary (in females) should be the norm. Sterilization procedures can and should be done without making disruptions to the endocrine system, which has long-term consequences for dogs.
- For dogs that have already been spayed or neutered, give them adrenal support with their food in the morning and thyroid support with their meal at night. If they eat once a day, combine these supplements.
- Do not feed dogs starch, sugar, unhealthy or cooked fats, and processed food. The dog's diet should be a carnivore diet with meat and bones.
- High glucose and high insulin are inflammatory in dogs. It is important to decrease them both.
- If changing to a Carnivore diet, then it must be done gradually, so the dog's digestive system can adjust.
- Dogs should intermittently fast throughout the week, or they can be fed one time a day.
- A healthy immune system is the key to fighting common diseases, such as cancer, because if the body creates this problem, then the body can fix this problem.
- Dogs need proactive treatment, not a treatment that is reactive to symptoms.
- Owners can stop cancer by increasing their dog's energy intake, metabolism, and immune system (through diet including protein, essential amino acids and fatty acids, minerals and vitamins).

- Treatment for a dog with cancer should include a proper diet and intermittent fasting.
- Owners and veterinarians should stop over vaccinating dogs.
- Antioxidants can help prevent disease while cytokine modulation, including blocking chemokines, will likely prove to be more promising for the future of improving the quality and longevity of your dog's life.
- A significant improvement for dog health can be achieved by following this basic tenant: health addition can be achieve by subtracting unhealthy food and artificial adverse exposures.

For more information, please refer to:

BaisavHealth.com

Global Health Science Solutions, LLC.

ChloeHealth.org

Bibliography

1. Adams, KM, AM Navarro, EK Hutchinson, and JL Weed. "A Canine Socialization and Training Program at the National Institutes of Health." *Lab Animal.* 33, no. 1 (January 2004): 32-36.

2. Ahlquist, R P, and B Levy. "Adrenergic Receptive Mechanisms of Canine Ileum." *Journal of Pharmacology Exp Ther* 127 (October 1959): 146–49.

3. Alho, Ana Margarida, José Meireles, Manuela Schnyder, Luís Cardoso, Silvana Belo, Peter Deplazes, and Luís Madeira De Carvalho. "Dirofilaria Immitis and Angiostrongylus Vasorum: The Current Situation of Two Major Canine Heartworms in Portugal." *Veterinary Parasitology* 252 (March 2018): 120–26. https://doi.org/10.1016/j.vetpar.2018.01.008.

4. "Aldosterone." Aldosterone | Endocrine Society, 2020. https://www.hormone.org/your-health-and-hormones/glands-and-hormones-a-to-z/hormones/aldosterone.

5. Aresu, L., P. Buracco, R. De Maria, S. Iussich, M. Martano, E. Morello, G. Bettini, S. Comazzi, F. Riondato, and L. Marconato. "'The Italian-Canine Cancer (ICC) Biobank: Our 10-Year Challenge,'" August 2019, 314–15. https://doi.org/10.1002/hon.2602/v2/response1.

6. Baghi, Hossein Bannazadeh, Ahad Bazmani, and Mohammad Aghazadeh. "Canine Vaccination: Bridging the Rabies Knowledge Gap." *Vaccine* 36, no. 1 (January 2, 2018): 4–5. https://doi.org/10.1016/j.vaccine.2017.11.016.

7. Baioni, Elisa, Eugenio Scanziani, Maria Claudia Vincenti, Mauro Leschiera, Elena Bozzetta, Marzia Pezzolato, Rosanna Desiato, Silvia Bertolini, Cristiana Maurella, and Giuseppe Ru. 2017. "Estimating Canine Cancer Incidence: Findings from a Population-Based Tumour Registry in Northwestern Italy." *BMC Veterinary Research* 13 (1): 203. https://doi.org/10.1186/s12917-017-1126-0.

8. Balogh, Orsolya, Rupert Bruckmaier, Stefanie Keller, and Iris Margaret Reichler. "Effect of Maternal Metabolism on Fetal Supply: Glucose, Non-Esterified Fatty Acids and Beta-Hydroxybutyrate Concentrations in Canine Maternal Serum and Fetal Fluids at Term Pregnancy." *Animal Reproduction Science* 193 (June 2018): 209–16. https://doi.org/10.1016/j.anireprosci.2018.04.072.

9. Bartges JW, CA Osborne, JP Lulich, JM Kruger, SL Sanderson, LA Koehler, and LK Ulrich. "Canine Urate Urolithiasis Etionathogenesis Diagnosis and Management." *Veterinary Clinic of North America. Small Animal Practice.* 29, no. 1 (January 1999). 161-91.

10. Bartner, L R, S McGrath, S Rao, L K Hyatt, and L A Wittenburg. "Pharmacokinetics of Cannabidiol Administered by 3 Delivery Methods at 2 Different Dosages to Healthy Dogs." *Canadian Journal of Veterinary Research* 82, no. 3 (July 2018): 178–83.

11. Bastidas, J.augusto, Michael J. Zinner, Jaime A. Bastidas, Marlene S. Orandle, and Charles J. Yeo. "Influence of Meal Composition on Canine Jejunal Water and Electrolyte Absorption." *Gastroenterology* 102, no. 2 (February 1992): 486–92. https://doi.org/10.1016/0016-5085(92)90094-f.

12. Beaulieu, A. D., J. K. Drackley, T. R. Overton, and L. S. Emmert. "Isolated Canine and Murine Intestinal Cells Exhibit a Different Pattern of Fuel Utilization for Oxidative Metabolism." *Journal of Animal Science* 80, no. 5 (May 2002): 1223–32. https://doi.org/10.2527/2002.8051223x.

13. Bednar, Geoff E., Avinash R. Patil, Sean M. Murray, Christine M. Grieshop, Neal R. Merchen, and George C. Fahey. "Starch and Fiber Fractions in Selected Food and Feed Ingredients Affect Their Small Intestinal Digestibility and Fermentability and Their Large Bowel Fermentability In Vitro in a Canine Mode." *The Journal of Nutrition* 131, no. 2 (January 2001): 276–86. https://doi.org/10.1093/jn/131.2.276.

14. Bermingham, Emma N., Paul Maclean, David G. Thomas, Nicholas J. Cave, and Wayne Young. "Key Bacterial Families (Clostridiaceae, Erysipelotrichaceae and Bacteroidaceae) Are Related to the Digestion of Protein and Energy in Dogs." *PeerJ* 5 (March 2, 2017). https://doi.org/10.7717/peerj.3019.

15. Berns, Gregory S., Andrew M. Brooks, and Mark Spivak. "Scent of the Familiar: An FMRI Study of Canine Brain Responses to Familiar and Unfamiliar Human and Dog Odors." *Behavioural Processes* 110 (January 2015): 37–46. https://doi.org/10.1016/j.beproc.2014.02.011.

16. Bischoff, Karyn, and Wilson K. Rumbeiha. "Pet Food Recalls and Pet Food Contaminants in Small Animals." *Veterinary Clinics of North America: Small Animal Practice* 42, no. 2 (November 2018): 237–50. https://doi.org/10.1016/j.cvsm.2011.12.007.

17. Boer, Benjamin De. "The Distribution Of Water And Fat In The Skin And Muscle Of The Dog During Chronic And Acute Dehydration." *American Journal of Physiology-Legacy Content* 147, no. 1 (September 1946): 49–53. https://doi.org/10.1152/ajplegacy.1946.147.1.49.

18. Boo, Gianluca, Stefan Leyk, Sara Irina Fabrikant, Andreas Pospischil, and Ramona Graf. "Assessing Effects of Structural Zeros on Models of Canine Cancer Incidence: a Case Study of the Swiss Canine Cancer Registry." *Geospatial Health* 12, no. 1 (May 11, 2017): 539. https://doi.org/10.4081/gh.2017.539.

19. Bouvet, J., C. Cariou, A. Poulard, F. Oberli, L. Cupillard, and P.m. Guigal. "Compatibility between a Rabies Vaccine and a Combined Vaccine against Canine Distemper, Adenovirosis, Parvovirosis, Parainfluenza Virus and Leptospirosis." *Veterinary Immunology and Immunopathology* 205 (November 2018): 93–96. https://doi.org/10.1016/j.vetimm.2018.11.001.

20. Bowman, D D, and J Drake. "Examination of the 'Susceptibility Gap' in the Treatment of Canine Heartworm Infection." *Parasite Vectors* 10 (November 2017): 513. https://doi.org/10.1186/s13071-017-2433-9.

21. Bree, Freek P J Van, Gertie C A M Bokken, Robin Mineur, Frits Franssen, Marieke Opsteegh, Joke W B Van Der Giessen, Len J A Lipman, and Paul A M Overgaauw. "Zoonotic Bacteria and Parasites Found in Raw Meat-Based Diets for Cats and Dogs." *Veterinary Record* 182, no. 2 (January 2018): 50–50. https://doi.org/10.1136/vr.104535.

22. Breheny, Craig R., Richard J. Mellanby, Julie A. Hamilton, and Adam G. Gow. "The Effect of Ammonia on Canine Polymorphonuclear Cells." *Veterinary Research Communications* 42, no. 3 (September 2018): 221–25. https://doi.org/10.1007/s11259-018-9725-1.

23. Bremhorst, Annika, Sarah Bütler, Hanno Würbel, and Stefanie Riemer. "Incentive Motivation in Pet Dogs – Preference for Constant vs Varied Food Rewards." *Scientific Reports* 8, no. 1 (June 27, 2018): 9756. https://doi.org/10.1038/s41598-018-28079-5.

24. Buff, P. R., R. A. Carter, J. E. Bauer, and J. H. Kersey. "Natural Pet Food: A Review of Natural Diets and Their Impact on Canine and Feline Physiology." *Journal of Animal Science* 92, no. 9 (January 2014): 3781–91. https://doi.org/10.2527/jas.2014-7789.

25. Bunford, Nóra, Vivien Reicher, Anna Kis, Ákos Pogány, Ferenc Gombos, Róbert Bódizs, and Márta Gácsi. "Differences in Pre-Sleep Activity and Sleep Location Are Associated with Variability in Daytime/Nighttime Sleep Electrophysiology in the Domestic Dog." *Scientific Reports* 8, no. 1 (August 2018). https://doi.org/10.1038/s41598-018-25546-x.

26. Burdett, S W, W D Mansilla, and A K Shoveller. "Many Canadian Dog.and Cat Foods Fail to Comply with the Guaranteed Analysis Reported on Packages." *Canadian Veterinary Journal* 59, no. 11 (November 2018): 1181–86.

27. Burri, Lena, Cathy Wyse, Stuart R. Gray, William S. Harris, and Kali Lazzerini. "Effects of Dietary Supplementation with Krill Meal on Serum pro-Inflammatory Markers after the Iditarod Sled Dog Race." *Research in Veterinary Science* 121 (December 2018): 18–22. https://doi.org/10.1016/j.rvsc.2018.10.002.

28. Butterwick, R. F., P. J. Markwell, and C. J. Thorne. "Effect of Level and Source of Dietary Fiber on Food Intake in the Dog." *The Journal of Nutrition* 124, no. 12 (December 1994). https://doi.org/10.1093/jn/124.suppl_12.2695s.

29. Butterwick, Richard F., and Amanda J. Hawthorne. "Advances in Dietary Management of Obesity in Dogs and Cats." *The Journal of Nutrition* 128, no. 12 (December 1998). https://doi.org/10.1093/jn/128.12.2771s.

30. Calogiuri, G, A Rossi, D Formenti, and A Weydahl. "Sleep Recovery in Participants After Racing in Finnmarkslop- Europe's Longest Sled-Dog Race." *Journal of Sports Medicine and Physical Fitness* 57, no. 1-2 (2017): 103–10. https://doi.org/10.23736/S0022-4707.16.05922-3.

31. Caren, Jf, Jh Meyer, and Mi Grossman. "Canine Intestinal Secretion during and after Rapid Distention of the Small Bowel." *American Journal of Physiology-Legacy Content* 227, no. 1 (July 1974): 183–88. https://doi.org/10.1152/ajplegacy.1974.227.1.183.

32. Cerbo, Alessandro Di, Julio Cesar Morales-Medina, Beniamino Palmieri, Federica Pezzuto, Raffaella Cocco, Gonzalo Flores, and Tommaso Iannitti. "Functional Foods in Pet Nutrition: Focus on Dogs and Cats." *Research in Veterinary Science* 112 (June 2017): 161–66. https://doi.org/10.1016/j.rvsc.2017.03.020.

33. Cersosimo, E., P. Williams, B. Hoxworth, W. Lacy, and N. Abumrad. "Glutamine Blocks Lipolysis and Ketogenesis of Fasting." *American Journal of Physiology-Endocrinology and Metabolism* 250, no. 3 (March 1986). https://doi.org/10.1152/ajpendo.1986.250.3.e248.

34. Chandler, Marjorie L., and Gregg Takashima. "Nutritional Concepts for the Veterinary Practitioner." *Veterinary Clinics of North America: Small Animal Practice* 44, no. 4 (July 2014): 645–66. https://doi.org/10.1016/j.cvsm.2014.03.009.

35. Charalambous, Marios. "Antiepileptic Drugs' Tolerability and Safety – a Systematic Review and Meta-Analysis of Adverse Effects in Dogs." *Veterinary Evidence* 1, no. 4 (May 2016): 79. https://doi.org/10.18849/ve.v1i4.83.

36. Chastant-Mailard, S, C Aggouri, A Albaret, A Eournier, and H Mila. "Canine and Feline Colostrum." *Reproduction in Domestic Animals.* 52, no. 2 (April 2017): 148-152.

37. Chen, Chi-Hung, Hsin-Bai Yin, Abhinav Upadhayay, Stephanie Brown, and Kumar Venkitanarayanan. "Efficacy of Plant-Derived Antimicrobials for Controlling Salmonella Schwarzengrund on Dry Pet Food." *International Journal of Food Microbiology* 296 (May 2019): 1–7. https://doi.org/10.1016/j.ijfoodmicro.2019.02.007.

38. Chikazawa, S., and M. D. Dunning. "A Review of Anaemia of Inflammatory Disease in Dogs and Cats." *Journal of Small Animal Practice* 57, no. 7 (July 2016): 348–53. https://doi.org/10.1111/jsap.12498.

39. Choi, Kyoungju, Maria T. Ortega, Brett Jeffery, Jim E. Riviere, and Nancy A. Monteiro-Riviere. "Oxidative Stress Response in Canine in Vitro Liver, Kidney and Intestinal Models with Seven Potential Dietary Ingredients." *Toxicology Letters* 241 (January 2016): 49–59. https://doi.org/10.1016/j.toxlet.2015.11.012.

40. Cima, G. "What's in Pet Food?" *Journal of American Veterinary Medical Association* 246, no. 10 (May 2015): 1028–33.

41. Clemmons, R M, R A Yamaguchi, R G Schaub, J Fleming, M R Dorsey-Lee, and T L McDonald. "1. Interaction between Canine Platelets and Adult Heartworms: Platelet Recognition of Heartworm Surfaces." *American Journal of Veterinary Research* 47, no. 2 (February 1986): 322–25.

42. Cochran, Donald R. "Walking My Dogs." *Journal of Palliative Medicine* 21, no. 11 (November 2018): 1665–65. https://doi.org/10.1089/jpm.2018.0161.

43. Coles, Tad B, and Michael W Dryden. 2014. "Insecticide/Acaricide Resistance in Fleas and Ticks Infesting Dogs and Cats." *Parasites & Vectors* 7 (1): 8. https://doi.org/10.1186/1756-3305-7-8.

44. Conway, Danielle M. P., and Korinn E. Saker. "Consumer Attitude Toward the Environmental Sustainability of Grain-Free Pet Foods." *Frontiers in*

Veterinary Science 5 (September 24, 2018): 170. https://doi.org/10.3389/fvets.2018.00170.

45. Cotman, C, E Head, B Muggenburg, S Zicker, and N Milgram. "Brain Aging in the Canine: a Diet Enriched in Antioxidants Reduces Cognitive Dysfunction." *Neurobiology of Aging* 23, no. 5 (2002): 809–18. https://doi.org/10.1016/s0197-4580(02)00073-8.

46. Craig, J. Mark. "Atopic Dermatitis and the Intestinal Microbiota in Humans and Dogs." *Veterinary Medicine and Science* 2, no. 2 (February 23, 2016): 95–105. https://doi.org/10.1002/vms3.24.

47. Creevy, KE, SN Austad, JM Hoffman, DG O'Neill, and DE Promislow. "The Companion Dog as a Model for the Longvity Dividend." *Cold Spring Harbor Perpectives in Medicine.* 6, no.1 (January 4, 2016).

48. Criswell, Theodore P., Matthew Macgregor Sharp, Howard Dobson, Ciara Finucane, Roy O. Weller, Ajay Verma, and Roxana O. Carare. "The Structure of the Perivascular Compartment in the Old Canine Brain: a Case Study." *Clinical Science* 131, no. 22 (November 13, 2017): 2737–44. https://doi.org/10.1042/cs20171278.

49. Cummings, Brian J., Elizabeth Head, William Ruehl, Norton W. Milgram, and Carl W. Cotman. "The Canine as an Animal Model of Human Aging and Dementia." *Neurobiology of Aging* 17, no. 2 (1996): 259–68. https://doi.org/10.1016/0197-4580(95)02060-8.

50. Davidson, Diana Ruth. "5 Dog Nose Facts You Probably Didn't Know." dog nose |, n.d. https://westsidedognanny.com/tag/dog-nose/.

51. Day, M.j. "Immune System Development in the Dog and Cat." *Journal of Comparative Pathology* 137 (July 2007). https://doi.org/10.1016/j.jcpa.2007.04.005.

52. Decaro, Nicola, and Canio Buonavoglia. "Canine Parvovirus Post-Vaccination Shedding: Interference with Diagnostic Assays and Correlation with Host Immune Status." *The Veterinary Journal* 221 (March 2017): 23–24. https://doi.org/10.1016/j.tvjl.2017.01.020.

53. De-Oliveira, L. D., M. A. De Carvalho Picinato, I. M. Kawauchi, N. K. Sakomura, and A. C. Carciofi. "Digestibility for Dogs and Cats of Meat and Bone Meal Processed at Two Different Temperature and Pressure Levels*." *Journal of Animal Physiology and Animal Nutrition* 96, no. 6 (December 29, 2011): 1136–46. https://doi.org/10.1111/j.1439-0396.2011.01232.x.

54. Desai, Rajiv. "Dr Rajiv Desai." Dr Rajiv Desai THE STRESS Comments, November 1, 2011. http://drrajivdesaimd.com/2011/11/01/the-stress/comment-page-10/.

55. "Digesting Bones, Gastric Acidity, Salmonella in Dogs and Cats." Vets All Natural, October 19, 2018. https://vetsallnatural.com.au/digesting-bones-gastric-acidity-salmonella-dogs-cats/?s=.

56. Dimakopoulos, Aristotelis C., and R. John Mayer. "Aspects of Neurodegeneration in the Canine Brain." *The Journal of Nutrition* 132, no. 6 (June 2002). https://doi.org/10.1093/jn/132.6.1579s.

57. Dodd, Sarah A. S., Nick J. Cave, Jennifer L. Adolphe, Anna K. Shoveller, and Adronie Verbrugghe. "Plant-Based (Vegan) Diets for Pets: A Survey of Pet Owner Attitudes and Feeding Practices." *Plos One* 14, no. 1 (January 2019). https://doi.org/10.1371/journal.pone.0210806.

58. "Dog Psychology – 10 Facts on How Your Dog's Mind Works." The Fabulous Dog Bed Company, May 17, 2018. https://www.thefabulousdogbedcompany.co.uk/blog/read_184273/dog-psychology-10-facts-on-how-your-dogs-mind-works.html.

59. Dong, Y, and H Hu. "Taming the 'Black Dog' by Light: A Retina-Habenula Circuit Mechanism Unveiled." *Neuron* 102, no. 1 (April 2019): 3–5. https://doi.org/10.1016/.neuron.2019.02.033.

60. Dowling, A L, and E Head. "Antioxidants in the Canine Model of Human Aging." *Biochim Biophys Acta* 1822, no. 5 (May 2012): 685–89. https://doi.org/10.1016/j.bbadis.2011.09.020.

61. Dzanis, David A. "Understanding Regulations Affecting Pet Foods." *Topics in Companion Animal Medicine* 23, no. 3 (August 2008): 117–20. https://doi.org/10.1053/j.tcam.2008.04.002.

62. Dzul-Rosado, Karla, Cesar Lugo-Caballero, Raul Tello-Martin, Karina López-Avila, and Jorge Zavala-Castro. 2017. "Direct Evidence of *Rickettsia Typhi* Infection in *Rhipicephalus Sanguineus* Ticks and Their Canine Hosts." *Open Veterinary Journal* 7 (2): 165–69. https://doi.org/10.4314/ovj.v7i2.14.

63. Erus, Nola. "Dog Tail Positions and What They Mean." BarkleyAndPaws, n.d. https://www.barkleyandpaws.com/dogs/health/dog-tail-positions-and-what-they-mean.

64. "Estrogen and Progesterone: Two Hormones That Control a Woman's Life." TAYLOR MEDICAL WELLNESS, WEIGHT LOSS AND AESTHETIC

GROUP, n.d. https://taylormedicalgroup.net/healthtopics/estrogen-and-progesterone.

65. "Explore Hormones,Observation, Treatment Details from Idea Clinics." Idea Clinics, 2020. https://www.ideaclinics.com/hormones-section/.

66. Farcus, A K, J A Larsen, T J Owens, R W Nelson, P H Kass, and A J Fascetti . "1. Management of Diabetes Melitus, Obesity, and Dietary Fat-Responsive Disease in Dogs." *Journal of American Veterinary Medicine Association* 257, no. 5 (September 2015): 501–7. https://doi.org/10.2460/javma.247.5.501.

67. Farcas, Amy K., Jennifer A. Larsen, and Andrea J. Fascetti. "Evaluation of Fiber Concentration in Dry and Canned Commercial Diets Formulated for Adult Maintenance or All Life Stages of Dogs by Use of Crude Fiber and Total Dietary Fiber Methods." *Journal of the American Veterinary Medical Association* 242, no. 7 (2013): 936–40. https://doi.org/10.2460/javma.242.7.936.

68. Fekete, S., Tibor Gaál, M. Hegedűs, F. Janza, and L. Zöldág. "Dog Feeding Test For Assessing The Nutritional Adequacy Of Practical Diets." *Acta Veterinaria Hungarica* 48, no. 1 (2000): 51–58. https://doi.org/10.1556/avet.48.2000.1.6.

69. Felsburg, P J. "Overview of Immune System Development in the Dog: Comparison with Humans." *Human & Experimental Toxicology* 21, no. 9-10 (2002): 487–92. https://doi.org/10.1191/0960327102ht286oa.

70. Ferguson, Glenn. "Comment on Canine Scent Detection for the Diagnosis of Lung Cancer in a Screening-like Situation." *Journal of Breath Research* 11, no. 3 (August 2017): 038001. https://doi.org/10.1088/1752-7163/aa78fe.

71. Fine, Adrian. "Effects of Acute Metabolic Acidosis on Renal, Gut, Liver, and Muscle Metabolism of Glutamine and Ammonia in the Dog." *Kidney International* 21, no. 3 (March 1982): 439–44. https://doi.org/10.1038/ki.1982.44.

72. Fleeman, L. M., and J.S. Rand. "Management of Canine Diaetes." *Veterinary Clinic of North America: Small Animal Practice.* 31, no. 5 (September 2001): 855-80.

73. Foster, Bethney. "Facts About Dogs' Brains." Facts About Dogs' Brains | Dog Care - Daily Puppy, n.d. https://dogcare.dailypuppy.com/dogs-brains-2711.html.

74. Gamble, L., A. D. Gibson, K. Shervell, F. Lohr, I. Otter, and R.j. Mellanby. "The Problem of Stray Dogs." *Revue Scientifique Et Technique De LOIE* 37, no. 2 (August 2018): 543–50. https://doi.org/10.20506/rst.37.2.2822.

75. Gamble, Lauri-Jo, Jordyn M. Boesch, Christopher W. Frye, Wayne S. Schwark, Sabine Mann, Lisa Wolfe, Holly Brown, Erin S. Berthelsen, and Joseph J. Wakshlag. "Pharmacokinetics, Safety, and Clinical Efficacy of Cannabidiol Treatment in Osteoarthritic Dogs." *Frontiers in Veterinary Science* 5 (July 2018). https://doi.org/10.3389/fvets.2018.00165.

76. Gardner, Heather L., Joelle M. Fenger, and Cheryl A. London. "Dogs as a Model for Cancer." *Annual Review of Animal Biosciences* 4, no. 1 (2016): 199–222. https://doi.org/10.1146/annurev-animal-022114-110911.

77. Gaykwad, C., J. Garkhal, G. E. Chethan, S. Nandi, and U. K. De. "Amelioration of Oxidative Stress UsingN-Acetylcysteine in Canine Parvoviral Enteritis." *Journal of Veterinary Pharmacology and Therapeutics* 41, no. 1 (February 2017): 68–75. https://doi.org/10.1111/jvp.12434.

78. Gentschev, Ivaylo, Sandeep Patil, Ivan Petrov, Joseph Cappello, Marion Adelfinger, and Aladar Szalay. "Oncolytic Virotherapy of Canine and Feline Cancer." *Viruses* 6, no. 5 (May 16, 2014): 2122–37. https://doi.org/10.3390/v6052122.

79. Gerencser, Linda, Nora Bunford, Alexandra Moesta, and Adam Miklosi. "Development and Validation of the Canine Reward Responsiveness Scale-Examining Individual Differences in Reward Responsiveness of the Domestic Dog." *Scientific Reports.* 8, no. 1 (March 13, 2018).

80. Gershwin, L.J. "Adverse Reactions to Vaccination: From Anaphylaxis to Autoimmunity." *Veterinary Clinic of North America: Small Animal Practice.* 48, no. 2 (March 2018): 279-90. https:// doi:10.1016/j.cvsm.2017.10.005.

81. Godoy, Maria R C De. "PANCOSMA COMPARATIVE GUT PHYSIOLOGY SYMPOSIUM: ALL ABOUT APPETITE REGULATION: Effects of Diet and Gonadal Steroids on Appetite Regulation and Food Intake of Companion animals1." *Journal of Animal Science* 96, no. 8 (July 28, 2018): 3526–36. https://doi.org/10.1093/jas/sky146.

82. Godoy, Maria De, Katherine Kerr, and Jr. George Fahey. "Alternative Dietary Fiber Sources in Companion Animal Nutrition." *Nutrients* 5, no. 8 (June 2013): 3099–3117. https://doi.org/10.3390/nu5083099.

83. Gomi, Hiroshi, Hiromi Osawa, Rie Uno, Tasdashi Yasui, Masahiro Hosaka, Seiji Torii, and Azuma Tsukise. "Canine Salivary Glands: Analysis of Rab and SNARE Protein Expression and SNARE Complex Formation with Diverse Tissue Properties." *Journal of Histochemistry & Cytochemistry.* 65, no. 11 (November 2017): 637-53.

84. Greene, Craig E., Ronald D. Schultz, and Richard B. Ford. "Canine Vaccination." *Veterinary Clinics of North America: Small Animal Practice* 31, no. 3 (May 2001): 473–92. https://doi.org/10.1016/s0195-5616(01)50603-8.

85. Groff, Katherine, and Patricia Bishop. 2017. "Itching for Change: Embracing Modern Flea and Tick Product Development." *Regulatory Toxicology and Pharmacology* 88 (August): 349–55. https://doi.org/10.1016/j.yrtph.2017.07.002.

86. Groothuis, Dennis R., Donald C. Wright, and Christoph B. Ostertag. "The Effect of 125I Interstitial Radiotherapy on Blood-Brain Barrier Function in Normal Canine Brain." *Journal of Neurosurgery* 67, no. 6 (December 1987): 895–902. https://doi.org/10.3171/jns.1987.67.6.0895.

87. Gross, Bill, David Garcia-Tapia, Elizabeth Riedesel, Norman Matthew Ellinwood, and Jackie K. Jens. "Normal Canine Brain Maturation At Magnetic Resonance Imaging." *Veterinary Radiology & Ultrasound* 51, no. 4 (2010): 361–73. https://doi.org/10.1111/j.1740-8261.2010.01681.x.

88. Grześkowiak, Łukasz, Akihito Endo, Shea Beasley, and Seppo Salminen. "Microbiota and Probiotics in Canine and Feline Welfare." *Anaerobe* 34 (August 2015): 14–23. https://doi.org/10.1016/j.anaerobe.2015.04.002.

89. Hackner, Klaus, and Joachim Pleil. "Canine Olfaction as an Alternative to Analytical Instruments for Disease Diagnosis: Understanding 'Dog Personality' to Achieve Reproducible Results." *Journal of Breath Research* 11, no. 1 (January 9, 2017): 012001. https://doi.org/10.1088/1752-7163/aa5524.

90. Hale, Ellen. "Canine Human-Scent-Matching: The Limitations of Systematic Pseudo Matching-to-Sample Procedures." *Forensic Science International* 279 (October 2017): 177–86. https://doi.org/10.1016/j.forsciint.2017.08.014.

91. Harper, EJ. "Changing Perspectives on Aging and Energy Requirements: Aging and Digestive Function in Humans, Dogs and Cats." *The Journal of Nutrition.* 128, no. 12(December 1998): 2928-35.

92. Harper, Tisha A.m. "Conservative Management of Hip Dysplasia." *Veterinary Clinics of North America: Small Animal Practice* 47, no. 4 (July 2017): 807–21. https://doi.org/10.1016/j.cvsm.2017.02.007.

93. Heanes, Dl. "Vitamin A Concentrations in Commercial Foods for Dogs and Cats." *Australian Veterinary Journal* 67, no. 8 (August 1990): 291–94. https://doi.org/10.1111/j.1751-0813.1990.tb07799.x.

94. Heilmann, Romy M., and Jörg M. Steiner. "Clinical Utility of Currently Available Biomarkers in Inflammatory Enteropathies of Dogs." *Journal of Veterinary Internal Medicine* 32, no. 5 (September 2018): 1495–1508. https://doi.org/10.1111/jvim.15247.

95. Hendricks, WH, EJ Bakker, and G Bosch. "Protein and Amino Acid Bioavailability Estimates for Canine Foods." *Journal of Animal Science.* 93, no. 10 (October 2015). 4788-95.

96. Hill, Richard C., Daniel D. Lewis, Karen C. Scott, Mayuko Omori, Melissa Jackson, Deborah A. Sundstrom, Galin L. Jones, John R. Speakman, Celeste A. Doyle, and Richard F. Butterwick. "Effect of Increased Dietary Protein and Decreased Dietary Carbohydrate on Performance and Body Composition in Racing Greyhounds." *American Journal of Veterinary Research* 62, no. 3 (March 2001): 440–47. https://doi.org/10.2460/ajvr.2001.62.440.

97. Hinder, R A, and K A Kelly. "Canine Gastric Emptying of Solids and Liquids." *American Journal of Physiology-Endocrinology and Metabolism* 233, no. 4 (January 1977): 335–40. https://doi.org/10.1152/ajpendo.1977.233.4.e335.

98. Hofmann, Rainer, Reynaldo Gomez, Emil A. Tanagho, and Jack W. Mcaninch. "Motility and Intraluminal Pressure of the Ileocolonic Junctional Zone and Adjacent Bowel in a Canine Model." *Urological Research* 21, no. 5 (1993): 329–32. https://doi.org/10.1007/bf00296830.

99. Holsapple, Michael P., Lori J. West, and Kenneth S. Landreth. "Species Comparison of Anatomical and Functional Immune System Development." *Birth Defects Research Part B: Developmental and Reproductive Toxicology* 68, no. 4 (August 2003): 321–34. https://doi.org/10.1002/bdrb.10035.

100. Holst, Bodil S., Malin H. Gustavsson, Anders Johannisson, Anna Hillström, Emma Strage, Ulf Olsson, Eva Axnér, and Inger Lilliehöök. "Inflammatory Changes during Canine Pregnancy." *Theriogenology* 125 (February 2019): 285–92. https://doi.org/10.1016/j.theriogenology.2018.11.016.

101. Holt, Rhonda L., Jana M. Gordon, and Craig Ruaux. "Immediate Effect of Transmucosal Application of Corn Syrup or 50% Dextrose Solution on Blood Glucose Concentrations in Healthy Dogs." *Journal of Veterinary Emergency and Critical Care* 29, no. 6 (2019): 630–34. https://doi.org/10.1111/vec.12897.

102. Horner, M. J., S. M. Ward, W. T. Gerthoffer, K. M. Sanders, and B. Horowitz. "Maintenance of Morphology and Function of Canine Proximal Colon Smooth Muscle in Organ Culture." *American Journal of Physiology-*

Gastrointestinal and Liver Physiology 272, no. 3 (January 1997). https://doi.org/10.1152/ajpgi.1997.272.3.g669.

103. Hooda, Seema, Yasushi Minamoto, Jan S. Suchodolski, and Kelly S. Swanson. "Current State of Knowledge: the Canine Gastrointestinal Microbiome." *Animal Health Research Reviews* 13, no. 1 (June 2012): 78–88. https://doi.org/10.1017/s1466252312000059.

104. "How Long Do You Leave Your Dog?" ArabianLines.Com Forum, August 21, 2010. http://arabianlines.com/forum1/topic_new.asp?TOPIC_ID=42190&whichpage=2.

105. Huang, H.-P., and Y.-H. Lien. "Effects of a Structured Exercise Programme in Sedentary Dogs with Chronic Diarrhoea." *Veterinary Record* 180, no. 9 (March 4, 2016): 224–24. https://doi.org/10.1136/vr.103902.

106. Jacobs, JA, JB Coe, DL Pearl, TM Widowski, and L Neil. "Factors Associated with Canine Resource Guarding Behavior in the Presence of People: A Cross-Sectional Survey of Dog Owners." *Preventative Veterinary Medicine.* 161, no. 1 (December 2018): 143-53.

107. Jasek, Judy. "FAQ's," February 19, 2020. https://rawdogfoodandco.com/transition-raw-dog-food/.

108. Jenkins, Eileen K., Mallory T. Dechant, and Erin B. Perry. "When the Nose Doesn't Know: Canine Olfactory Function Associated With Health, Management, and Potential Links to Microbiota." *Frontiers in Veterinary Science* 5 (March 29, 2018): 56. https://doi.org/10.3389/fvets.2018.00056.

109. Jensen, Kristine B., and Daniel L. Chan. "Nutritional Management of Acute Pancreatitis in Dogs and Cats." *Journal of Veterinary Emergency and Critical Care* 24, no. 3 (2014): 240–50. https://doi.org/10.1111/vec.12180.

110. Jergens, Albert E. "Inflammatory Bowel Disease in Veterinary Medicine." *Frontiers in Bioscience* E4, no. 4 (January 2012): 1404–19. https://doi.org/10.2741/e470.

111. Kallfelz, F A. "Nutrition and Feeding of Dogs and Cats. Past, Present, and Future. ." *Cornell Vet* 75, no. 1 (January 1985): 221–29.

112. Kanakubo, Kayo, Andrea J. Fascetti, and Jennifer A. Larsen. "Assessment of Protein and Amino Acid Concentrations and Labeling Adequacy of Commercial Vegetarian Diets Formulated for Dogs and Cats." *Journal of the American Veterinary Medical Association* 247, no. 4 (August 15, 2015): 385–92. https://doi.org/10.2460/javma.247.4.385.

113. Keef, K. D., S. M. Ward, R. J. Stevens, B. W. Frey, and K. M. Sanders. "Electrical and Mechanical Effects of Acetylcholine and Substance P in Subregions of Canine Colon." *American Journal of Physiology-Gastrointestinal and Liver Physiology* 262, no. 2 (January 1992). https://doi.org/10.1152/ajpgi.1992.262.2.g298.

114. Kehoe, Siobhan. "Why Do Dogs Hear Better than Humans?" HeadStuff, March 31, 2015. https://www.headstuff.org/topical/science/dogs-hear-better-humans/.

115. Kerby, Justin. "When Is the Best Time to Drink Coffee? (According to Science)." Cave Social, November 28, 2018. https://www.cavesocial.com/the-best-time-to-drink-coffee-according-to-science/.

116. Killick, D. R., A. J. Stell, and B. Catchpole. "Immunotherapy for Canine Cancer - Is It Time to Go Back to the Future?" *Journal of Small Animal Practice* 56, no. 4 (April 2015): 229–41. https://doi.org/10.1111/jsap.12336.

117. Kimmel, Susan E., Kathryn E. Michel, Rebecka S. Hess, and Cynthia R. Ward. "Effects of Insoluble and Soluble Dietary Fiber on Glycemic Control in Dogs with Naturally Occurring Insulin-Dependent Diabetes Mellitus." *Journal of the American Veterinary Medical Association* 216, no. 7 (2000): 1076–81. https://doi.org/10.2460/javma.2000.216.1076.

118. Kis, Anna, Anna Gergely, Ágoston Galambos, Judit Abdai, Ferenc Gombos, Róbert Bódizs, and József Topál. "Sleep Macrostructure Is Modulated by Positive and Negative Social Experience in Adult Pet Dogs." *Proceedings of the Royal Society B: Biological Sciences* 284, no. 1865 (October 25, 2017): 20171883. https://doi.org/10.1098/rspb.2017.1883.

119. Kogan, Lori, Regina Schoenfeld-Tacher, Peter Hellyer, and Mark Rishniw. "US Veterinarians Knowledge, Experience, and Perception Regarding the Use of Cannabidiol for Canine Medical Conditions." *Frontiers in Veterinary Science* 5 (January 2019). https://doi.org/10.3389/fvets.2018.00338.

120. Konno, Akitsugu, Miho Inoue-Murayama, Shinji Yabuta, Akiko Tonoike, Miho Nagasawa, Kazutaka Mogi, and Takefumi Kikusui. "Effect of Canine Oxytocin Receptor Gene Polymorphism on the Successful Training of Drug Detection Dogs." *Journal of Heredity* 109, no. 5 (June 2018): 566–72. https://doi.org/10.1093/jhered/esy012.

121. Kozlowska, Kasia, Peter Walker, Loyola Mclean, and Pascal Carrive. "Fear and the Defense Cascade." *Harvard Review of Psychiatry* 23, no. 4 (2015): 263–87. https://doi.org/10.1097/hrp.0000000000000065.

122. Kramer, L., S. Crosara, G. Gnudi, M. Genchi, C. Mangia, A. Viglietti, and C. Quintavalla. "Wolbachia, Doxycycline and Macrocyclic Lactones: New Prospects in the Treatment of Canine Heartworm Disease." *Veterinary Parasitology* 254 (April 2018): 95–97. https://doi.org/10.1016/j.vetpar.2018.03.005.

123. Kranz, William, Kelley Kitts, Nicholas Strange, Joshua Cummins, Erica Lotspeich, and John Goodpaster. "On the Smell of Composition C-4." *Forensic Science International* 236 (March 2014): 157–63. https://doi.org/10.1016/j.forsciint.2013.12.012.

124. Kruis, W., A. Haddad, and S.f. Phillips. "Chenodeoxycholic and Ursodeoxycholic Acids Alter Motility and Fluid Transit in the Canine Ileum." *Digestion* 34, no. 3 (1986): 185–95. https://doi.org/10.1159/000199328.

125. Kruis, W., F. Azpiroz, and S. F. Phillips. "Contractile Patterns and Transit of Fluid in Canine Terminal Ileum." *American Journal of Physiology-Gastrointestinal and Liver Physiology* 249, no. 2 (August 1985). https://doi.org/10.1152/ajpgi.1985.249.2.g264.

126. Kuchitsu, Yoshihiko, Yuta Homma, Naonobu Fujita, and Mitsunori Fukuda. "Rab7 Knockout Unveils Regulated Autolysosome Maturation Induced by Glutamine Starvation." *Journal of Cell Science* 131, no. 7 (April 7, 2018). https://doi.org/10.1242/jcs.215442.

127. Kunze, Christopher P., James J. Hoskinson, Michael D. Butine, and Justin M. Goggin. "Evaluation Of Solid Phase Radiolabels Of Dog Food For Gastric Emptying." *Veterinary Radiology Ultrasound* 40, no. 2 (1999): 169–73. https://doi.org/10.1111/j.1740-8261.1999.tb01904.x.

128. Larson, J A, and A Farcas. "Nutrition of Aging Dogs." *Veterinary Clinic of North America: Small Animal Practice* 44 (July 2014): 741–59. https://doi.org/10.1016/j.cvsm.

129. Lavan, Robert, Rob Armstrong, Kaan Tunceli, and Dorothy Normile. "Dog Owner Flea/Tick Medication Purchases in the USA." *Parasites & Vectors* 11, no. 1 (November 6, 2018): 581. https://doi.org/10.1186/s13071-018-3142-8.

130. Lea, Stephen E. G., and Britta Osthaus. "In What Sense are Dogs Special? Canine Cognition in Comparative Context." *Learning & Behavior.* 46, no. 4 (December 2018): 335-63.

131. Leclerc, Lucie, Chantal Thorin, John Flanagan, Vincent Biourge, Samuel Serisier, and Patrick Nguyen. "Higher Neonatal Growth Rate and Body

Condition Score at 7 Months Are Predictive Factors of Obesity in Adult Femal Beagle Dogs." *BMC Veterinary Research*. 13, no. 1 (2017). https://doi.org/10.1186/s12917-017-0994-7.

132. Lemieux, Guy, Patrick Vinay, Gabriel Baverel, Raymond Brière, and André Gougoux. "Relationship between Lactate and Glutamine Metabolism in Vitro by the Kidney: Differences between Dog and Rat and Importance of Alanine Synthesis in the Dog." *Kidney International* 16, no. 4 (October 1979): 451–58. https://doi.org/10.1038/ki.1979.150.

133. Leonard, Jayne. "Hypothyroidism Symptoms: 12 Signs to Look out For." Medical News Today. MediLexicon International, February 25, 2019. https://www.medicalnewstoday.com/articles/324535.

134. Lepor, Herbert, James Mohler, Mary Baumann, and Ellen Shapiro. "Comparison of Muscarinic Cholinergic and Alpha Adrenergic Receptors in Canine Ileum, Colon, Intestinal Urinary Reservoirs and Bladder." *Journal of Urology* 142, no. 1 (July 1989): 204–8. https://doi.org/10.1016/s0022-5347(17)38711-6.

135. Levine, Corri B., Julie Bayle, Vincent Biourge, and Joseph J. Wakshlag. "Effects and Synergy of Feed Ingredients on Canine Neoplastic Cell Proliferation." *BMC Veterinary Research* 12, no. 1 (August 2, 2016): 159. https://doi.org/10.1186/s12917-016-0774-9.

136. Li, Qinghong, Christian L. Lauber, Gail Czarnecki-Maulden, Yuanlong Pan, and Steven S. Hannah. "Effects of the Dietary Protein and Carbohydrate Ratio on Gut Microbiomes in Dogs of Different Body Conditions." *MBio* 8, no. 1 (January 24, 2017). https://doi.org/10.1128/mbio.01703-16.

137. Linder, Deborah E., and Valerie J. Parker. "Dietary Aspects of Weight Management in Cats and Dogs." *Veterinary Clinics of North America: Small Animal Practice* 46, no. 5 (2016): 869–82. https://doi.org/10.1016/j.cvsm.2016.04.008.

138. Mainardi, L. "Niacin, Niacinamide and Blood Sugar." *Acta Vitaminol Enzymol* 21, no. 4 (n.d.): 139–59.

139. Maloney, A. H., Beverly Graves, and L. Cecil Rhodes. "Carbohydrate Metabolism During Prolonged Ether and Chloroform Anesthesia." *Anesthesia & Analgesia* 28, no. 1 (1949). https://doi.org/10.1213/00000539-194901000-00018.

140. Maria, A. P. J., L. Ayane, T. C. Putarov, B. A. Loureiro, B. P. Neto, M. F. Casagrande, M. O. S. Gomes, M. B. A. Glória, and A. C. Carciofi. "The Effect of Age and Carbohydrate and Protein Sources on Digestibility, Fecal Microbiota, Fermentation Products, Fecal IgA, and Immunological Blood Parameters in Dogs." *Journal of Animal Science* 95, no. 6 (2017): 2452. https://doi.org/10.2527/jas2016.1302.

141. Martin, Guy, and Gabriel Baverel. "Lactate, Alanine and Glutamine Metabolism in Isolated Canine Pup Liver Cells." *Biochimica Et Biophysica Acta (BBA) - General Subjects* 760, no. 2 (October 1983): 230–37. https://doi.org/10.1016/0304-4165(83)90168-x.

142. Marx, FR, L Trevizan, FMBO Saad, KG Lisenko, JS Reis, and AM Kessler. "Endogenous Fat Loss and True Total Tract Digestibility of Poultry Fat in Adult Dogs." *Journal of Animal Science.* 95, no. 7 (July 2017): 2928-35.

143. Matousek, Jennifer L., Karen L. Campbell, Ibulaimu Kakoma, and David J. Schaeffer. "The Effects of Four Acidifying Sprays, Vinegar, and Water on Canine Cutaneous PH Levels." *Journal of the American Animal Hospital Association* 39, no. 1 (2003): 29–33. https://doi.org/10.5326/0390029.

144. McGetrick,Jand F Range. "Inequity Aversion in Dogs: A Review." *Learning & Behavior.* 46, no. 4 (December 2018): 479-500.

145. Mcgill, Erin, Olaf Berke, Andrew S. Peregrine, and J. Scott Weese. "Epidemiology of Canine Heartworm (Dirofilaria Immitis) Infection in Domestic Dogs in Ontario, Canada: Geographic Distribution, Risk Factors and Effects of Climate." *Geospatial Health* 14, no. 1 (May 13, 2019). https://doi.org/10.4081/gh.2019.741.

146. Mcgrath, Stephanie, Lisa R. Bartner, Sangeeta Rao, Rebecca A. Packer, and Daniel L. Gustafson. "Randomized Blinded Controlled Clinical Trial to Assess the Effect of Oral Cannabidiol Administration in Addition to Conventional Antiepileptic Treatment on Seizure Frequency in Dogs with Intractable Idiopathic Epilepsy." *Journal of the American Veterinary Medical Association* 254, no. 11 (June 2019): 1301–8. https://doi.org/10.2460/javma.254.11.1301.

147. Miller, Benjamin F., Sarah E. Ehrlicher, Joshua C. Drake, Frederick F. Peelor, Laurie M. Biela, Shannon L. Pratt-Phillips, Michael undefined Davis, and Karyn undefined Hamilton. "Assessment of Protein Synthesis in Highly Aerobic Canine Species at the Onset and during Exercise Training." *Journal of Applied Physiology* 118, no. 7 (April 1, 2015): 811–17. https://doi.org/10.1152/japplphysiol.00982.2014.

148. Miller, Eric J., Anne J. Gemensky-Metzler, David A. Wilkie, Rachel M. Wynne, Elizabeth M. Curto, and Heather L. Chandler. "Effects of Grape Seed Extract, Lutein, and Fish Oil on Responses of Canine Lens Epithelial Cells in

Vitro." *American Journal of Veterinary Research* 79, no. 7 (July 2018): 770–78. https://doi.org/10.2460/ajvr.79.7.770.

149. Mirimi, Rona. "The Importance of Estrogen and Progesterone." Fertility Aware, February 24, 2020. https://fertilityaware.co.za/the-importance-of-estrogen-and-progesterone/.

150. Mitchell, Cassie M., Brenda M. Davy, Matthew W. Hulver, Andrew P. Neilson, Brian J. Bennett, and Kevin P. Davy. "Does Exercise Alter Gut Microbial Composition? A Systematic Review." *Medicine & Science in Sports & Exercise* 51, no. 1 (January 2019): 160–67. https://doi.org/10.1249/mss.0000000000001760.

151. Mitchell, Judy A., and Joe Brownlie. "The Challenges in Developing Effective Canine Infectious Respiratory Disease Vaccines." *Journal of Pharmacy and Pharmacology* 67, no. 3 (March 2015): 372–81. https://doi.org/10.1111/jphp.12380.

152. Morelli, G., G. Marchesini, B. Contiero, E. Fusi, M. Diez, and R. Ricci. "A Survey of Dog Owners' Attitudes toward Treats." *Journal of Applied Animal Welfare Science* 23, no. 1 (17, 2019): 1–9. https://doi.org/10.1080/10888705.2019.1579095.

153. Motta, Luca, Maria Teresa Mandara, and Geoffrey C. Skerritt. "Canine and Feline Intracranial Meningiomas: An Updated Review." *The Veterinary Journal* 192, no. 2 (May 2012): 153–65. https://doi.org/10.1016/j.tvjl.2011.10.008.

154. Murray, SM, GC Fahey Jr, NR Merchen, GD Sunvol, and GA Reinhart. "Evaluation of Selected High-Starch Flours as Ingredients in Canine Diets." *Journal of Animal Science.* 77 no. 8 (October 2015): 2180-86.

155. Nagasawa, M, S Mitsui, S En, N Ohtani, M Ohta, Y Sakuma, T Onaka, K Mogi, and T Kikusui. "Social Evolution. Oxytocin-gaze Positive Loop and the Coevolution of Human Dog-Breeds." *Science.* 348 (April 17, 2015): 333-36.

156. Narvaes, Rodrigo, and Rosa Maria Martins De Almeida. "Aggressive Behavior and Three Neurotransmitters: Dopamine, GABA, and Serotonin—A Review of the Last 10 Years." *Psychology & Neuroscience* 7, no. 4 (2014): 601–7. https://doi.org/10.3922/j.psns.2014.4.20.

157. "Neurotranmitters Implicated in Dog Aggression." K9aggression.com, 2020. https://k9aggression.com/neurotranmitters-implicated-dog-aggression/?v=f24485ae434a.

158. Nishino, Seiji, Janis Arrigoni, Jeff Shelton, Takashi Kanbayashi, William C. Dement, and Emmanuel Mignot. "Effects of Thyrotropin-Releasing Hormone and Its Analogs on Daytime Sleepiness and Cataplexy in Canine Narcolepsy." *The Journal of Neuroscience* 17, no. 16 (August 15, 1997): 6401–8. https://doi.org/10.1523/jneurosci.17-16-06401.1997.

159. Nishzono, A. "Rabies." *Brain Nerve*, February 2009, 135–44.

160. Nixon, Sophie L., Lindsay Rose, and Annika T. Muller. "Efficacy of an Orally Administered Anti-Diarrheal Probiotic Paste (Pro-Kolin Advanced) in Dogs with Acute Diarrhea: A Randomized, Placebo-Controlled, Double-Blinded Clinical Study." *Journal of Veterinary Internal Medicine* 33, no. 3 (May 2019): 1286–94. https://doi.org/10.1111/jvim.15481.

161. "Nutritional Management in Dogs and Cats." *Veterinary Record* 178, no. 17 (April 2016): 427. https://doi.org/10.1136/vr.i2287. .

162. Nuttall, Danielle, Richard Butterwick, Katja Strauhs, and Phil Mcgenity. "Comparison of Measured and Predicted Energy Density of an Oral Care Chew for Dogs." *Journal of Nutritional Science* 6 (2017). https://doi.org/10.1017/jns.2017.24.

163. Ochiai, T. "Effects of Stress on Colon in the Canine." *Nihon Shakakibyo Gakkai Zasshi (The Japanese Journal of Gastro-Enterology).* 87, no 4 (April 1990): 965-72.

164. Olivry, Thierry, and Frane Banovic. "Treatment of Canine Atopic Dermatitis: Time to Revise Our Strategy?" *Veterinary Dermatology* 30, no. 2 (April 2019): 87–90. https://doi.org/10.1111/vde.12740.

165. Olivry, Thierry, and Ralf S. Mueller. "Critically Appraised Topic on Adverse Food Reactions of Companion Animals (5): Discrepancies between Ingredients and Labeling in Commercial Pet Foods." *BMC Veterinary Research* 14, no. 1 (2018). https://doi.org/10.1186/s12917-018-1346-y.

166. Olivry, Thierry, Jennifer Bexley, and Isabelle Mougeot. "Extensive Protein Hydrolyzation Is Indispensable to Prevent IgE-Mediated Poultry Allergen Recognition in Dogs and Cats." *BMC Veterinary Research* 13, no. 1 (August 17, 2017): 251. https://doi.org/10.1186/s12917-017-1183-4.

167. Otranto, Domenico. "Arthropod-Borne Pathogens of Dogs and Cats: From Pathways and Times of Transmission to Disease Control." *Veterinary Parasitology* 251 (February 2018): 68–77. https://doi.org/10.1016/j.vetpar.2017.12.021.

168. Overk, B, Svete A Nemec, J Salobir, V Rezar, and Petric A Domanjko. "Markers of Oxidative Stress in Dogs Wit Heart Failure." *Journal of Vererinary*

Diagn Invest, September 2017, 636–44. https://doi.org/10.1177/1040638717711995.

169. Ozawa, Makiko, Mai Inoue, Kazuyuki Uchida, James K. Chambers, Yukari Takeuch, and Hiroyuki Nakayama. "Physical Signs of Canine Cognitive Dysfunction." *Journal of Veterinary Medical Science* 81, no. 12 (December 2019): 1829–34. https://doi.org/10.1292/jvms.19-0458.

170. Pan, Yuanlong, Adam D. Kennedy, Thomas J. Jönsson, and Nortan W. Milgram. "Cognitive Enhancement in Old Dogs from Dietary Supplementation with a Nutrient Blend Containing Arginine, Antioxidants, B Vitamins and Fish Oil." *British Journal of Nutrition* 119, no. 3 (October 2018): 349–58. https://doi.org/10.1017/s0007114517003464.

171. Pawar, Mahesh M., Ashok K. Pattanaik, Dharmendra K. Sinha, Tapas K. Goswami, and Kusumakar Sharma. "Effect of Dietary Mannanoligosaccharide Supplementation on Nutrient Digestibility, Hindgut Fermentation, Immune Response and Antioxidant Indices in Dogs." *Journal of Animal Science and Technology* 59, no. 1 (May 11, 2017): 11. https://doi.org/10.1186/s40781-017-0136-6.

172. Pfister, Kurt, and Rob Armstrong. 2016. "Systemically and Cutaneously Distributed Ectoparasiticides: a Review of the Efficacy against Ticks and Fleas on Dogs." *Parasites & Vectors* 9 (1): 436. https://doi.org/10.1186/s13071-016-1719-7.

173. Ponglowhapan, Suppawiwat, Birgitta Essén-Gustavsson, and Catharina Linde Forsberg. "Influence of Glucose and Fructose in the Extender during Long-Term Storage of Chilled Canine Semen." *Theriogenology* 62, no. 8 (2004): 1498–1517. https://doi.org/10.1016/j.theriogenology.2004.02.014.

174. Poo-Muñoz, Daniela A., Claudia Elizondo-Patrone, Luis E. Escobar, Francisca Astorga, Sergio E. Bermúdez, Constanza Martínez-Valdebenito, Katia Abarca, and Gonzalo Medina-Vogel. 2016. "Fleas and Ticks in Carnivores From a Domestic–Wildlife Interface: Implications for Public Health and Wildlife." *Journal of Medical Entomology* 53 (6): 1433–43. https://doi.org/10.1093/jme/tjw124.

175. Post, Joseph M., and Joseph R. Hume. "Ionic Basis for Spontaneous Depolarizations in Isolated Circular Smooth Muscle Cells of the Canine Colon." *Gastroenterology* 103, no. 4 (1992): 1393. https://doi.org/10.1016/0016-5085(92)91624-d.

176. Poupko, Jay M., William Lee Hearn, and Federico Rossano. "Drug Contamination of U.S. Paper Currency and Forensic Relevance of Canine Alert to Paper Currency: A Critical Review of the Scientific Literature." *Journal of Forensic Sciences* 63, no. 5 (September 2018): 1340–45. https://doi.org/10.1111/1556-4029.13755.

177. Prins, Nicolaas H., Michel R. Briejer, and Jan A.j. Schuurkes. "Characterization of the Contraction to 5-HT in the Canine Colon Longitudinal Muscle." *British Journal of Pharmacology* 120, no. 4 (1997): 714–20. https://doi.org/10.1038/sj.bjp.0700954.

178. Puurunen, Jenni, Katriina Tiira, Katariina Vapalahti, Marko Lehtonen, Kati Hanhineva, and Hannes Lohi. "Fearful Dogs Have Increased Plasma Glutamine and γ-Glutamyl Glutamine." *Scientific Reports* 8, no. 1 (October 29, 2018): 15976. https://doi.org/10.1038/s41598-018-34321-x.

179. Queiroz, R. W., V. L. Silva, D. R. Rocha, D. S. Costa, S. H. N. Turco, M. T. B. Silva, A. A. Santos, M. B. L. Oliveira, A. S. R. Pereira, and R. C. Palheta-Junior. "Changes in Cardiovascular Performance, Biochemistry, Gastric Motility and Muscle Temperature Induced by Acute Exercise on a Treadmill in Healthy Military Dogs." *Journal of Animal Physiology and Animal Nutrition* 102, no. 1 (February 2018): 122–30. https://doi.org/10.1111/jpn.12667.

180. Rastall, R. A. "Bacteria in the Gut: Friends and Foes and How to Alter the Balance." *The Journal of Nutrition* 134, no. 8 (August 2004). https://doi.org/10.1093/jn/134.8.2022s.

181. Redfern, Alana, Jan Suchodolski, and Albert Jergens. "Role of the Gastrointestinal Microbiota in Small Animal Health and Disease." *Veterinary Record* 181, no. 14 (October 2017): 370–70. https://doi.org/10.1136/vr.103826.

182. Rialland, Pascale, Sylvain Bichot, Maxim Moreau, Martin Guillot, Bertrand Lussier, Dominique Gauvin, Johanne Martel-Pelletier, Jean-Pierre Pelletier, and Eric Troncy. "Clinical Validity of Outcome Pain Measures in Naturally Occurring Canine Osteoarthritis." *BMC Veterinary Research* 8, no. 1 (2012): 162. https://doi.org/10.1186/1746-6148-8-162.

183. Risio, Luisa De, Sofie Bhatti, Karen Muñana, Jacques Penderis, Veronika Stein, Andrea Tipold, Mette Berendt, et al. "International Veterinary Epilepsy Task Force Consensus Proposal: Diagnostic Approach to Epilepsy in Dogs." *BMC Veterinary Research* 11, no. 1 (August 28, 2015). https://doi.org/10.1186/s12917-015-0462-1.

184. Roccabianca, Paola. 2018. "Canine Skin Cancer and the Art of Classifications." *Veterinary Pathology* 55 (6): 770–71. https://doi.org/10.1177/0300985818790783.

185. Romanucci, Mariarita, and Leonardo Della Salda. "Oxidative Stress and Protein Quality Control Systems in the Aged Canine Brain as a Model for Human Neurodegenerative Disorders." *Oxidative Medicine and Cellular Longevity* 2015 (2015): 1–8. https://doi.org/10.1155/2015/940131.

186. Rose, L., J. Rose, S. Gosling, and M. Holmes. "Efficacy of a Probiotic-Prebiotic Supplement on Incidence of Diarrhea in a Dog Shelter: A Randomized, Double-Blind, Placebo-Controlled Trial." *Journal of Veterinary Internal Medicine* 31, no. 2 (March 2017): 377–82. https://doi.org/10.1111/jvim.14666.

187. Roudebush, Philip, Deborah J Davenport, and Bruce J Novotny. "The Use of Nutraceuticals in Cancer Therapy." *Veterinary Clinics of North America: Small Animal Practice* 34, no. 1 (2004): 249–69. https://doi.org/10.1016/j.cvsm.2003.09.001.

188. Roy, Meenakshi, Namshin Kim, Kyung Kim, Won-Hyong Chung, Rujira Achawanantakun, Yanni Sun, and Robert Wayne. "Analysis of the Canine Brain Transcriptome with an Emphasis on the Hypothalamus and Cerebral Cortex." *Mammalian Genome* 24, no. 11-12 (December 8, 2013): 484–99. https://doi.org/10.1007/s00335-013-9480-0.

189. Rybicka, Agata, and Magdalena Król. "Identification and Characterization of Cancer Stem Cells in Canine Mammary Tumors." *Acta Veterinaria Scandinavica* 58, no. 1 (December 2016): 86. https://doi.org/10.1186/s13028-016-0268-6.

190. Rychel, Jessica K. "Diagnosis and Treatment of Osteoarthritis." *Topics in Companion Animal Medicine* 25, no. 1 (February 2010): 20–25. https://doi.org/10.1053/j.tcam.2009.10.005.

191. Saalmüller, Armin. "New Understanding of Immunological Mechanisms." *Veterinary Microbiology* 117, no. 1 (October 2006): 32–38. https://doi.org/10.1016/j.vetmic.2006.04.007.

192. Sabatino, Daria Di, Giovanni Savini, and Alessio Lorusso. "Canine Distemper and Endangered Wildlife: Is It Time for Mandatory Vaccination of Dogs?" *Vaccine* 33, no. 48 (November 2015): 6519. https://doi.org/10.1016/j.vaccine.2015.05.087.

193. Saker, Korinn E. "Nutrition and Immune Function." *Veterinary Clinics of North America: Small Animal Practice* 36, no. 6 (November 2006): 1199–1224. https://doi.org/10.1016/j.cvsm.2006.09.001.

194. Sanchis-Mora, Sandra, Ludovic Pelligand, Holger A. Volk, and Siobhan M. Abeyesinghe. "Diagnosis and Treatment of Canine Neuropathic Pain." *Veterinary Record* 177, no. 18 (November 2015): 470. https://doi.org/10.1136/vr.h5927.

195. Satyaraj, E. "Emerging Paradigms in Immunonutrition." *Topics in Companion Animal Medicine.* 26, no. 1 (February 2011): 25-32.

196. Schiffman, Joshua D., and Matthew Breen. 2015. "Comparative Oncology: What Dogs and Other Species Can Teach Us about Humans with Cancer." *Philosophical Transactions of the Royal Society B: Biological Sciences* 370 (1673): 20140231. https://doi.org/10.1098/rstb.2014.0231.

197. Schmidt, Milena, Stefan Unterer, Jan S. Suchodolski, Julia B. Honneffer, Blake C. Guard, Jonathan A. Lidbury, Jörg M. Steiner, Julia Fritz, and Petra Kölle. "The Fecal Microbiome and Metabolome Differs between Dogs Fed Bones and Raw Food (BARF) Diets and Dogs Fed Commercial Diets." *Plos One* 13, no. 8 (August 2018). https://doi.org/10.1371/journal.pone.0201279.

198. Schmitz, Silke, and Jan Suchodolski. "Understanding the Canine Intestinal Microbiota and Its Modification by pro-, Pre- and Synbiotics - What Is the Evidence?" *Veterinary Medicine and Science* 2, no. 2 (January 11, 2016): 71–94. https://doi.org/10.1002/vms3.17.

199. Schoenfeld-Tacher, Regina M., Timothy J. Horn, Tyler A. Scheviak, Kenneth D. Royal, and Lola C. Hudson. "Evaluation of 3D Additively Manufactured Canine Brain Models for Teaching Veterinary Neuroanatomy." *Journal of Veterinary Medical Education* 44, no. 4 (2017): 612–19. https://doi.org/10.3138/jvme.0416-080r.

200. Schultz, Ronald D. "Duration of Immunity for Canine and Feline Vaccines: A Review." *Veterinary Microbiology* 117, no. 1 (October 2006): 75–79. https://doi.org/10.1016/j.vetmic.2006.04.013.

201. Sechi, S, F Fiore, C Dimauro, A Nudda, and R Cocco. "Oxidative Stress and Food Supplementation with Antioxidants in Therapy Dogs." *Canadian Journal of Veterinary Research* 81, no. 3 (July 2017): 206–16.

202. Seksel, Kersti. "Puppy Socialization Classes." *The Veterinary Clinics of North America: Small Animal Practice.* 27, no. 3 (May 1997):465-77.

203. Siegle, M. L., and H. J. Ehrlein. "Digestive Motor Patterns and Transit of Luminal Contents in Canine Ileum." *American Journal of Physiology-Gastrointestinal and Liver Physiology* 254, no. 4 (April 1988): 552–29. https://doi.org/10.1152/ajpgi.1988.254.4.g552.

204. Siegle, M. L., S. Buhner, M. Schemann, H. R. Schmid, and H. J. Ehrlein. "Propagation Velocities and Frequencies of Contractions along Canine Small Intestine." *American Journal of Physiology-Gastrointestinal and Liver Physiology* 258, no. 5 (May 1990): 738–44. https://doi.org/10.1152/ajpgi.1990.258.5.g738.

205. Simpson, BS. "Canine Comminication." *The Veterinary Clinics of North America: Small Animal Practice.* 27, no. 3 (May 1997): 445-64.

206. Sirek, Otakar V., and Charles H. Best. "Anterior Pituitary Growth Hormone and Blood Sugar Levels of Normal and Diabetic Dogs." *American Journal of Physiology-Legacy Content* 185, no. 3 (January 1956): 557–63. https://doi.org/10.1152/ajplegacy.1956.185.3.557.

207. Sleight, Douglas R., and Neil R. Thomford. "Gross Anatomy of the Blood Supply and Biliary Drainage of the Canine Liver." *The Anatomical Record* 166, no. 2 (1970): 153–60. https://doi.org/10.1002/ar.1091660204.

208. Smith, Allen D., Kiran S. Panickar, Joseph F. Urban, and Harry D. Dawson. "Impact of Micronutrients on the Immune Response of Animals." *Annual Review of Animal Biosciences* 6, no. 1 (2018): 227–54. https://doi.org/10.1146/annurev-animal-022516-022914.

209. Smith, Annette N. "The Role of Neutering in Cancer Development." *Veterinary Clinics of North America: Small Animal Practice* 44, no. 5 (September 2014): 965–75. https://doi.org/10.1016/j.cvsm.2014.06.003.

210. Smith, Robert J., and Douglas W. Wilmore. "Glutamine Nutrition and Requirements." *Journal of Parenteral and Enteral Nutrition* 14, no. 4_suppl (1990): 94–99. https://doi.org/10.1177/014860719001400412.

211. "Sniffer Dogs to Help Combat Wildlife Crime." *Veterinary Record* 183, no. 12 (September 29, 2018): 370–71. https://doi.org/10.1136/vr.k4089.

212. "Sniffer Dogs Unleashed." *Veterinary Record* 182, no. 14 (April 7, 2018): 394–95. https://doi.org/10.1136/vr.k1533.

213. Snigdha, Shikha, Christina De Rivera, Norton W. Milgram, and Carl W. Cotman. "Effect of Mitochondrial Cofactors and Antioxidants Supplementation on Cognition in the Aged Canine." *Neurobiology of Aging* 37 (January 2016): 171–78. https://doi.org/10.1016/j.neurobiolaging.2015.09.015.

214. Spinato, MT, IK Barker, and DM Houston. "A Morphometric Study of the Canine Colon: Comparison of Control Dogs and Cases of Colonic Disease." *Canadian Journal of Veterinary Research.* 54 , no. 4 (October 1990). 477-86.

215. Squires, Richard A. "Vaccines in Shelters and Group Settings." *Veterinary Clinics of North America: Small Animal Practice* 48, no. 2 (March 2018): 291–300. https://doi.org/10.1016/j.cvsm.2017.10.006.

216. Stahlmann, R, S Kuhner, M Shakibaei, J Flores, J Vormann, and DC van Sickle. "Effects of Magnesium Defiency on Joint Cartilage in Immature Beagle Dogs: Immunohistochemistry, Electron Microscopy, and Mineral Concentrations." *Archives of Toxicology.* 73, no. 10 (January 2000): 573-80.

217. Stephens, Jack. "4 Dog Facial Expressions and What They Mean." Pet Insurance Blog - Pets Best Insurance, September 6, 2019. https://www.petsbest.com/blog/4-dog-facial-expressions/?CI=5000002&spJobID=1282884924&spMailingID=55376158&spReportId=MTI4Mjg4NDkyNAS2&spUserID=MTcyMDc4MzM1MDI4S0&utm_campaign=Newsletter&utm_medium=email&utm_source=PHS

218. Stephens-Brown, Lara, and Michael Davis. "Water Requirements of Canine Athletes during Multi-Day Exercise." *Journal of Veterinary Internal Medicine* 32, no. 3 (May 2018): 1149–54. https://doi.org/10.1111/jvim.15091.

219. Streeter, Elizabeth M., Erika Zsombor-Murray, Kari E. Moore, John E. Rush, Jorg M. Steiner, Elizabeth A. Rozanski, Kathryn E. Michel, David A. Williams, and Lisa M. Freeman. "Intestinal Permeability and Absorption in Dogs with Traumatic Injury." *Journal of Veterinary Internal Medicine* 16, no. 6 (2002): 669–73. https://doi.org/10.1111/j.1939-1676.2002.tb02406.x.

220. Strompfová, Viola, Andrea Lauková, and Dušan Cilik. "Synbiotic Administration of Canine-Derived Strain Lactobacillus Fermentum CCM 7421 and Inulin to Healthy Dogs." *Canadian Journal of Microbiology* 59, no. 5 (May 2013): 347–52. https://doi.org/10.1139/cjm-2012-0472.

221. Strompfová, Viola, Ivana Kubašová, and Andrea Lauková. "Health Benefits Observed after Probiotic Lactobacillus Fermentum CCM 7421 Application in Dogs." *Applied Microbiology and Biotechnology* 101, no. 16 (August 18, 2017): 6309–19. https://doi.org/10.1007/s00253-017-8425-z.

222. Swanson, K S, C M Grieshop, G M Clapper, R G Shields, T Belay, N R Merchen, and G C Fahey. "Fruit and Vegetable Fiber Fermentation by Gut Microflora from Canines." *Journal of Animal Science* 79, no. 4 (2001): 919. https://doi.org/10.2527/2001.794919x.

223. Takahashi, Yasuro, Shigemitsu Ebihara, Yoshiko Nakamura, and Kiyohisa Takahashi. "A Model of Human Sleep-Related Growth Hormone Secretion in Dogs: Effects of 3, 6, and 12 Hours of Forced Wakefulness on Plasma Growth

Hormone, Cortisol, and Sleep Stages*." *Endocrinology* 109, no. 1 (July 1981): 262–72. https://doi.org/10.1210/endo-109-1-262.

224. Tanabe, Atsushi, Daisuke Kobayashi, Koki Maeda, Masayuki Taguchi, and Hiroeki Sahara. 2018. "Angiogenesis-Related Gene Expression Profile in Clinical Cases of Canine Cancer." *Veterinary Medicine and Science* 5 (1): 19–29. https://doi.org/10.1002/vms3.127.

225. Terlizzi, Roberta Di, and Simon Platt. "The Function, Composition and Analysis of Cerebrospinal Fluid in Companion Animals: Part I – Function and Composition." *The Veterinary Journal* 172, no. 3 (November 2006): 422–31. https://doi.org/10.1016/j.tvjl.2005.07.021.

226. "Test 1 A&P 2 ENDOCRINE & BLOOD." Quizlet, 2020. https://quizlet.com/333893352/test-1-ap-2-endocrine-blood-diagram/.

227. "The Problem with Starchy Foods. What Does This Mean for Veg in a Raw Diet?" Cotswold RAW, September 17, 2016. https://www.cotswoldraw.com/blog-headlines/the-problem-with-starchy-foods-what-does-this-mean-for-veg-in-a-raw-diet/.

228. Thielke, LE, and MA Udell. "The Role of Oxytocin in Relationships Between Dogs and Humans and Potential Applications for the Treatment of Separation Anxiety in Dogs." *Biological Reviews of the Cambridge Philosophical Society.* 92, no. 1 (Februaru 2017): 378-88.

229. Thomas, Richard K. "Non-Demographic Factors Associated with Morbidity." SpringerLink. Springer, New York, NY, December 19, 2015. https://link.springer.com/chapter/10.1007/978-1-4939-3423-2_6.

230. Thompson, H, and N.G. Wright. "Canine Salmonellosis." *The Journal of Small Animal Practice.* 1-, no. 10 (December 1969): 579-82.

231. Tjernsbekk, M. T., A.-H. Tauson, O. F. Kraugerud, and Ø. Ahlstrøm. "Raw Mechanically Separated Chicken Meat and Salmon Protein Hydrolysate as Protein Sources in Extruded Dog Food: Effect on Protein and Amino Acid Digestibility." *Journal of Animal Physiology and Animal Nutrition* 101, no. 5 (March 2017). https://doi.org/10.1111/jpn.12608.

232. Trevino, Jose Francisco, and Craig Marianno. "Calculation of Canine Dose Rate Conversion Factors for Photons and Electrons." *Health Physics* 114, no. 1 (January 2018): 20–26. https://doi.org/10.1097/hp.0000000000000732.

233. Tryfondidou, MA, MS Holl, MA Oosterlaken-Dijksterhuis, MVastenburg, WE van den Brom, and HA Hazewinkel. "Growth Hormone Modulates Cholecalciferol Metabolism with Moderate Effects on Intestinal Mineral

Absorption and Specific Effects on Bone Formation in Growing Dogs Raised on Balanced Food." *Domestic Animal Endocrimology.* 25, no. 2 (August 2003): 155-74.

234. Udell, Monique A. R. "A New Approach to Understanding Canine Social Cognition." *Learning & Behavior* 46, no. 4 (June 2018): 329–30. https://doi.org/10.3758/s13420-018-0334-1.

235. Vajdovich, Peter. "Free Radicals and Antioxidants in Inflammatory Processes and Ischemia-Reperfusion Injury." *Veterinary Clinics of North America: Small Animal Practice* 38, no. 1 (January 2008): 31–123. https://doi.org/10.1016/j.cvsm.2007.11.008.

236. Vannucchi, Ci, D Kishi, Fm Regazzi, Lcg Silva, Gal Veiga, Dsr Angrimani, Cf Lucio, and M Nichi. "The Oxidative Stress, Antioxidant Profile and Acid-Base Status in Preterm and Term Canine Neonates." *Reproduction in Domestic Animals* 50, no. 2 (April 2015): 240–46. https://doi.org/10.1111/rda.12476.

237. Venturini, K. S., M. F. Sarcinelli, M. A. Baller, T. C. Putarov, E. B. Malheiros, and A. C. Carciofi. "Processing Traits and Digestibility of Extruded Dog Foods with Soy Protein Concentrate." *Journal of Animal Physiology and Animal Nutrition* 102, no. 4 (November 2018): 1077–87. https://doi.org/10.1111/jpn.12894.

238. Vinod, Ashwin, John Staughton, Rujuta Pradhan, and Salama Yusuf. "Why Are Dogs So Good At Smelling Things?" Science ABC, November 14, 2019. https://www.scienceabc.com/nature/animals/why-dogs-sense-of-smell-is-so-good.html.

239. Wackermannová, M., L. Pinc, and L. Jebavý. "Olfactory Sensitivity in Mammalian Species." *Physiological Research* 65, no. 3 (July 18, 2016): 369–90. https://doi.org/10.33549/physiolres.932955.

240. Walden, Kat. "What Part of the Dog Brain Affects Behavior?" What Part of the Dog Brain Affects Behavior? | Dog Care - Daily Puppy, n.d. https://dogcare.dailypuppy.com/part-dog-brain-affects-behavior-5807.html.

241. Weese, J. "Oxalate Degradation by Intestinal Lactic Acid Bacteria in Dogs and Cats." *Veterinary Microbiology* 101, no. 3 (July 2004): 161–66. https://doi.org/10.1016/s0378-1135(04)00105-1.

242. Weidner, Nicole, and Adronie Verbrugghe. "Current Knowledge of Vitamin D in Dogs." *Critical Reviews in Food Science and Nutrition* 57, no. 18 (December 2016): 3850–59. https://doi.org/10.1080/10408398.2016.1171202.

243. Weidner, S, A Probst, and S Kneissl. "MR Anatomy of Salivary Glands in the Dog." *Anatomia, Histologia, Embryologia.* 41, no. 2. (April 2012):149-53.

244. Welch, Jeffrey. "7 Amazing Facts About Your Dog's Sense of Smell." 7 Amazing Facts About Your Dog's Sense of Smell, February 21, 2019. http://jeffreyrwelch.blogspot.com/2019/02/7-amazing-facts-about-your-dogs-sense.html.

245. While, Alison. "Pet Dogs as Promoters of Wellbeing." *British Journal of Community Nursing* 22, no. 7 (July 2, 2017): 332–36. https://doi.org/10.12968/bjcn.2017.22.7.332.

246. Yam, Philippa S., Gregory Naughton, Christina F. Butowski, and Amanda L. Root. "Inaccurate Assessment of Canine Body Condition Score, Bodyweight, and Pet Food Labels: A Potential Cause of Inaccurate Feeding." *Veterinary Sciences* 4, no. 4 (June 9, 2017): 30. https://doi.org/10.3390/vetsci4020030.

247. Zenoble, RD, and RJ Kemppainen. "Adrenocortical Suppression by Topically Applied Corticosteroids in Healthy Dogs." *Journal of the American Veterinary Medical Association.* 191, no. 6 (September 1987): 685-88.

248. Zheng, TZ, JJ Zheng, and YM Ma. "The Relationship Between Changes in Concentration of Blood Sugar and Period of Interdigestive 14 Myoelectric Complex." *Sheng Li Xue Bao* 43, no. 6 (December 1991): 584-588.

Acknowledgement

A Message from Chloe: Dogs are Not Cows

A special tribute to Chloe, our British Cream Golden Retriever, with a portion of the proceeds going to dog shelters as Chloe's act of kindness resonates as a sounding board for dog health.

I would like to thank Chloe's immediate family, Danielle, Bailey, and Savannah Willette, and extended family, my mother, Enola A. Willette, and father, Charles E Willette, and the rest of the family, Debbie, Chuckie and John Willette.

A special thanks to Benefactors: Lois and Bob Santoro, Jenny and Tom Hauser, Carol and Ray Stephens, and Madalyn Martin

Thank you to artist/ medical illustrator Jade Panyko and graphic designer Skaila Angulo.

Finally, a special thanks to Atlantic Publishing Group, Inc., founder Mr. Doug Brown, and consultant Mr. Jack Bissell.

Lastly, a special thanks to editor Kassandra White.

A heart felt thank you to all.

Paul M. Willette MD
Global Health Science Solutions LLC.
Website BaisavHealth.com

www.ingramcontent.com/pod-product-compliance
Lightning Source LLC
Chambersburg PA
CBHW070927270326
41927CB00011B/2749